Traumatic Stress in South Africa

Traumatic Stress in South Africa

Debra Kaminer and Gillian Eagle

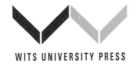

WITS UNIVERSITY PRESS

Wits University Press
1 Jan Smuts Avenue
Johannesburg
2001
South Africa
http://witspress.ac.za

First published 2010

ISBN 978-1-86814-509-6

Edited by Lara Jacob
Indexed by Ethné Clarke
Cover design by Hybridcreative
Layout by Manoj Sookai
Printed and bound by Creda Communications

Wits University Press has made every reasonable effort to locate, contact and acknowledge copyright owners. Please notify us should copyright not have been properly identified and acknowledged. Any corrections will be incorporated in subsequent editions of the book.

Cover: *Blue Head, 1993* by William Kentridge

The authors are deeply grateful for the thoughtful and reflective comments provided by colleagues, friends and loved ones during the preparation of this book.

TABLE OF CONTENTS

LIST OF ABBREVIATIONS AND ACRONYMS

ANC	African National Congress
ASD	Acute Stress Disorder
BPP	Brief Psychodynamic Psychotherapy
CBT	Cognitive Behavioural Therapy
CIDI	Composite International Diagnostic Interview
CISD	Critical Incident Stress Debriefing
CPT	Cognitive Processing Therapy
CSVR	Centre for the Study of Violence and Reconciliation
CT	Cognitive Therapy
DESNOS	Disorders of extreme stress not otherwise specified
EA	Employee Assistance
EMDR	Eye Movement Desensitisation and Reprocessing
IFP	Inkatha Freedom Party
IRCT	International Rehabilitation Council for Torture Victims
MVAs	Motor vehicle accidents
NGOs	Non-governmental organisations
NLP	Neurolinguistic Programming

NPAT	National Peace Accord Trust
PE	Prolonged Exposure
PIE	Proximity, Immediacy and Expectancy
POWA	People Opposing Women Abuse
PSTD	Posttraumatic Stress Disorder
PTGI	Post Traumatic Growth Inventory
SADF	South African Defence Force
SANDF	South African National Defence Force
SASH	South African Stress and Health
SIT	Stress Inoculation Training
SSRIs	Selective serotonin reuptake inhibitors
TFT	Thought Field Therapy
TIR	Traumatic Incident Reduction
TRC	Truth and Reconciliation Commission
VKD	Visual Kinaesthetic Dissociation

Chapter 1

INTRODUCTION

The aim of this book is to address the pressing and socially relevant topic of traumatic stress in South Africa. Given the high levels of exposure to trauma and violence of various kinds in this country, there is naturally serious concern about the mental health impact and implications of this exposure.

South African citizens are widely and commonly confronted with anecdotal accounts of traumatic events, both in the course of their everyday lives and in the mass media, often articulated in the discourse of living in a dangerous and traumatised society. Along with this awareness of the frequent occurrence of trauma is a preoccupation with its psychological consequences. The notion of 'posttraumatic stress' has entered the public domain to the extent that this terminology is in common usage and is even used to describe the state of characters in popular local television dramas or 'soap operas'. It is also noticeable that in media accounts of traumatic events there are frequently references to the fact that victims are receiving debriefing or counselling, suggesting that trauma intervention is offered by many practitioners of various levels of skill to large numbers of trauma survivors, with an assumption that such intervention should take place as a matter of course. The increasing awareness of and prominence given to posttraumatic stress conditions and related interventions has had benefits and costs. Although the public may be better informed about some aspects of traumatic stress and victims may more readily access and seek assistance, there are also misconceptions and problematic practices. Common sense or folkloric knowledge of traumatic stress can easily become dated, distorted or misinterpreted. Access to up-to-date, well substantiated and clearly presented information about traumatic stress is important at this point in time, both in terms of doing justice to the international advancements in traumatic stress knowledge and in terms of improving everyday practices in South Africa. In response to this need, this book presents an overview of aspects of trauma prevalence, impact and treatment that is intended to be both scholarly and accessible. This text aims to be mindful of the complexities of working with trauma survivors living within a context of multiple dangers.

Although the term *trauma* is often associated with medical conditions, as in physical trauma to the body, this book focuses on psychological trauma or trauma to the psyche. The origin of the word *trauma* lies in a Greek word meaning 'to tear' or 'to puncture'[1]. In the case of psychological trauma this understanding is reflected in a notion of psychological wounding and the penetration of unwanted thoughts, emotions and experiences into the psyche or being of the person. Traumatic experiences are usually unanticipated and by definition place excessive demands on people's existing coping strategies. Thus traumatic events create severe disruptions to many aspects of psychological functioning.

The term 'trauma' has been used to refer both to stimuli of a catastrophic nature ('the assault was a trauma in her life') and to the severe distress produced by such an event ('she experienced trauma as a consequence of the assault'), and in this book it is similarly used to refer to both events and responses. As will become clearer in the later discussion of the impact of trauma, this dual meaning perhaps makes sense when one appreciates that trauma is characterised by the coupling of a dreadful experience with a subjective experience of dread – the outcome and its cause are inextricably intertwined. In this respect *traumatic* stress is a very specific type of stress, distinguishable from other forms of stress by the severity of both the stressor and the response. The study of traumatic stress is a distinct field of theory and research with some overlap with the stress field, but with a largely independent conceptual base and orientation. The field of traumatic stress (or traumatology as it is sometimes referred to) encompasses a broad range of issues and has generated a substantial body of psychological writing, particularly since the 1970s, with ever-widening interest.

In South Africa, psychological interest in traumatic stress has specific origins which have to some extent shaped the kinds of knowledge generated here. For many South Africans working as both researchers and interventionists in the traumatic stress field, interest in the phenomenon was generated out of a 'political' investment. Whether this investment had its origins in anti-apartheid resistance politics or was informed by commitment to a general human rights agenda, many South African trauma researchers and practitioners have been drawn to the field out of moral, rather than purely academic, concerns. Much of the early work in the trauma field in South Africa, reflected in writing from the 1970s and 1980s, was not conceived of necessarily as falling under the umbrella of 'traumatic stress'. For example, during this period traumatic stress terminology was not widely employed in discussions of the work of the volunteer-based Rape Crisis and People Opposing Women Abuse (POWA) organisations or the work of therapists providing support to ex-detainees and torture survivors. Nevertheless, in hindsight, it is apparent that the activist work engaged in by sub-groups of psychologists, doctors, volunteer counsellors and other mental health practitioners was indeed traumatic stress intervention and contributed to the initial observation and documentation of traumatic stress phenomena in this country. As the diagnosis of posttraumatic stress and related conditions became popularised in the United States and internationally, the domain of traumatic stress studies became better defined and constructs from within this repertoire became more widely employed in South Africa. Also, with political change, the study of traumatic stress became open to more purely academic interests. However, the activist origins that shaped the early generation of knowledge in this field have been retained to some extent. As much of the case material and empirical research cited in this book reflects, looking at society through the lens of traumatic stress highlights social problems and relations of oppression. Indeed, as the American psychiatrist and feminist activist Judith Herman noted, 'to hold traumatic reality in consciousness requires a social context that affirms and protects the victim and that joins victim and witness in a common alliance'.[2] Engaging with traumatised individuals means taking on board the origins of their plight and this may well entail a profound comprehension of abuses and inequities in society. Whether as an academic or a practitioner, working in the trauma field requires engagement with the relationship between personal and social ills. Thus it is still possible to align research and activist interests in studying trauma, even if the political context has changed.

South Africa's history of political violence coupled with its contemporary high rates of violent crime, sexual and domestic violence and road accident injury (amongst other issues), has unfortunately meant that the country represents, in some ways, 'a natural laboratory' in which to study the impact of traumatic events and their consequences. Changes in the social fabric of South African society tend to be reflected in shifts in the focus of traumatic stress research, with researchers engaging with new issues and populations of interest in order to stay abreast of contemporary historical developments. For example, there is currently a strong interest in the interface between HIV- and AIDS-related issues and aspects of traumatic stress. New social agendas constantly replace those of the past, although some issues, such as the problem of sexual violence, seem to endure.

While there are clearly broader debates informing the trauma field, such as those concerning the causes of endemic interpersonal violence in South Africa and appropriate strategies for preventing traumatisation, the focus of this particular text is on the topic of trauma itself, with a thorough examination of trauma prevalence, impact and intervention. While recognising that the causes and consequences of trauma cannot always be easily separated, it is the latter that is of primary interest in this text, together with a range of other aspects of traumatisation.

Over time there has been increasing formalisation in the execution and documentation of research related to traumatic stress in South Africa. Although there are still enormous gaps in the knowledge base concerning traumatic stress in this country, there is increasing investment in both quantitative and qualitative research. Perhaps because early trauma interventionists prioritised social activism over publishing, little of this work was documented in formal academic texts and journals. Rather, knowledge was captured in the form of manuals, minutes of meetings and congress proceedings. Much of this material lies untapped as a historical record of early trauma work in South Africa. In addition, there is also a large body of knowledge held within current non-governmental organisations (NGOs) that is slowly becoming increasingly more rigorously documented and presented. While there has been a very strong interest in traumatic stress research across a number of South African universities in the last two decades, much of this research has been captured in the form of student research projects, masters theses and doctorates and has not been published and widely disseminated beyond this. Within this book we attempt to draw upon a wide a range of sources of knowledge in order to provide as rich a picture of the traumatic stress terrain in the country as we can. However, one of the strands running through the various chapters is the need for more directed research and research publication in a range of areas, as well as the need for increased integration of knowledge across the field. One of the important contributions of this book is that it offers a cohesive picture of trauma prevalence, impact and intervention in South Africa and in this respect provides a unique synthesis of existing knowledge.

Although this book has a strong focus on South African issues, it is not parochial in its outlook. The text covers seminal international work in the trauma domain as well as contemporary international debates and up-to-date research. The international traumatic stress research field is rich and vibrant and the book aims to reflect this, while also using a critical lens to evaluate the relevance of the international traumatic stress knowledge base for South African conditions. While the implications of trauma theory for the South African context are unpacked, South African phenomena that have potential to contribute to international theorisation are also highlighted. Although South African concerns are not necessarily unique to this setting, there are contextually driven trauma imperatives that require innovation in theorisation and intervention. South African society is marked by high levels of exposure to traumatic events, the likelihood of multiple exposure and the possibility of re-exposure to such events, and by constraints in trauma intervention accessibility and availability. In addition, trauma takes place against a backdrop of extreme wealth disparities, powerful race sensitivities and cultural hybridity. Trauma theorists and practitioners have grappled with, and continue to explore, the implications of these local trauma characteristics for the presentation of traumatic stress conditions and optimal intervention. Engagement with some of these issues is a major aim of this book.

Having provided some broad background to the book, the main content will be briefly described so as to orientate the reader. Chapter 2, which follows, provides a picture of the scope of the problem of trauma exposure in South Africa. The prevalence of different kinds of trauma is reviewed, and the specific populations in South Africa who are most at risk for experiencing different forms of trauma are highlighted. Comparison is made to international literature on rates and patterns of trauma exposure, and some of the gaps and difficulties in accurately assessing local prevalence rates are noted. In Chapter 3 the mental health impact of traumatic events is presented, with a particular focus on the formally diagnosable condition of Posttraumatic Stress Disorder (PTSD).[3] The symptoms and dysfunction associated with PTSD and related conditions are discussed, with some emphasis on the fact that victims or survivors of trauma may present with a range of mental health problems beyond PTSD. Some critiques of the diagnostic perspective are also raised. The chapter concludes with a synthesis of South African research on the impact of trauma. In Chapter 4 the discussion of the impact of trauma is broadened to include a focus on the disruption of the survivor's meaning systems and what this entails for psychological adjustment. Individual and contextual influences on meaning-making are emphasised. Chapter 5 then moves on to look at some of the mechanisms for addressing the impact of psychological trauma, with a primary focus on various forms of psychotherapeutic intervention for individual survivors. Group and community initiatives are also considered, as well as some particular issues raised by working in the South African context. In Chapter 6 much of the broad material covered previously in the book is revisited, but with a particular focus on children. Issues pertaining to the prevalence, impact and treatment of traumatic stress in the child and adolescent population in South Africa are explored. Finally, in Chapter 7, some overarching thoughts on the nature of trauma in South Africa and possible future directions for trauma research are offered. We trust you will find the coverage stimulating and the book engaging to read.

Chapter 2

PATTERNS OF TRAUMA EXPOSURE IN SOUTH AFRICA

The South African media is consistently filled with local stories of crime, violence and injury. Internationally, too, South Africa has an increasingly dubious reputation as a highly dangerous place. But are these images of South Africa supported by objective, systematic evidence? Just how dangerous is our society when compared with other countries? What forms of trauma and violence pose the greatest burden to our society? And is South Africa equally dangerous for everyone?

Certainly, South Africa is one of the few countries in the world that has endured protracted political violence as well as high rates of criminal violence, domestic abuse and accidental injury. This translates into a large number of trauma survivors in our society, with one nationally representative survey reporting that 75 per cent of respondents had experienced a traumatic event in their lifetime and over half had experienced multiple traumas.[1] The same study also established that there are many South Africans who have not experienced a trauma directly, but have been indirectly traumatised through the sudden death of a loved one, hearing about a trauma that occurred to a person they are close to, or witnessing a traumatic incident. It is therefore apparent that very few South Africans live lives completely untouched by trauma and, for many, exposure to potentially traumatic experiences is an inescapable part of daily life.

While no one in South Africa is immune from trauma, some people are more at risk than others of experiencing certain kinds of trauma. Understanding the prevalence of different forms of trauma in the population is an important first step in developing strategies to reduce the burden of trauma in our society. This chapter will review patterns of exposure to the most common forms of violence and accidental injury, as well as indirect and multiple trauma exposure.

Violence

As is the case elsewhere in the world, gender is a strong predictor of whether or not South Africans will be exposed to a particular form of violence. As we shall see, certain types of violence in South Africa are more likely to occur to women and others are more likely to affect men. Beginning in 2002, the South African Stress and Health (SASH) study conducted a survey of trauma exposure in a nationally representative sample of 4,351 South African adults.[2] The rates of exposure to different forms of violence that were reported by men and women in the SASH survey are presented in Table 2.1. Each of these forms of violence exposure will now be considered in some detail.

Political violence

Politically motivated human rights abuses are a feature of many socio-political systems worldwide. Amnesty International has documented the commission of human rights violations such as abductions, torture, genocide and detention without trial in 153 countries, with victims numbering in the hundreds of thousands.[3] Although political violence is no longer a common feature of South African society, many South Africans have survived the political violence that characterised the apartheid era. During the apartheid years, the South African state consistently denied or minimised rates of state-perpetrated violence, and it was only as the South African Truth and Reconciliation Commission (TRC) process unfolded in the mid-1990s that the levels of political violence to which South Africans had been exposed truly became clear.

Table 2.1
Prevalence of exposure to different forms of violence in a nationally representative sample of South African adults

	Males (%)	Females (%)	Total (%)
Political violence			
Severe ill-treatment	2.7**	0.6	1.6
Detention	2.4**	0.3	1.3
Torture	1.3**	0.2	0.7
Criminal violence	25.9**	11.6	18.2
Gender-based violence			
Physical abuse by intimate partner	1.3	13.6**	7.9
Rape	0.3	3.7 **	2.1
Other sexual assault	1.0	2.1*	1.6
Physical abuse during childhood	12.3	11.7	12.0

Significantly higher level than counterpart at p < 0.05 level
**Significantly higher level than counterpart at p < 0.0001 level*
Source: Kaminer et al., 2008

According to the evidence collected by the TRC, forms of political violence and traumatisation that were particularly common in South Africa during apartheid included the political detention and torture of those who were active in the anti-apartheid struggle, the abduction and murder of suspected political activists, stoning, shooting and beating of people engaged in political protests, and the intentional destruction of homes and property.[4] As the TRC noted in its final report, these forms of political violence were carried out by members of the state security forces in an attempt to suppress anti-apartheid activity, and the victims of these forms of violence were primarily black South Africans.[5] In particular, male youths were most commonly the victims of organised state violence, since they were often on the 'front lines' of the struggle against apartheid. And in the final years of apartheid, possibly as the result of provocation by state security forces, there was also a high level of violence between different political factions in black townships, again affecting mostly male youths.

Detention without trial was the most pervasive form of repression carried out by the South African state during the apartheid years. Political detention could be an extremely traumatic experience, not only because the conditions in detention were very harsh, but also because apartheid security laws meant that detention could go on indefinitely. Many South Africans were detained for up to three years without trial. In the SASH survey, 2.4 per cent of men and 0.3 per cent of women reported that they had been detained under apartheid security laws, indicating that, today, many tens of thousands of South Africans are ex-detainees. The vast majority of detainees were young men, but, between 1960 and 1990, some 10,000 women and 15,000 children younger than fifteen years old were also detained.[6]

Many of those who were detained during apartheid were subjected to torture, for the purposes of obtaining information or a confession and punishing the person for suspected anti-apartheid activities.[7] According to testimonies given to the TRC by torture survivors, the forms of torture employed by South African security forces included beatings, electric shocks, suffocation, drowning, deprivation of food and sleep, exposure to the elements, forced posture and excessive physical exercise, attacks by dogs and sexual abuse. In addition, many forms of psychological torture were used, such as falsely telling a detainee that a family member or comrade was dead, forcing a detainee to observe the torture of a fellow detainee, and emotional humiliation and degradation. Over 5,000 incidents of torture were reported to the TRC by about 3,000 people, mainly concerning the violation of black men between the ages of thirteen and thirty-six years old.[8] In the more recent nationally representative SASH survey, 1.3 per cent of men and 0.2 percent of women in the sample reported having been tortured,[9] a statistic which suggests that several thousand South Africans have survived torture. But these figures probably represent only a minority of all torture experiences in the South African population. It is possible that some torture survivors in South Africa, as in other countries, have never revealed their torture experiences to anyone, due to a deep sense of shame and humiliation, feelings of guilt for having given evidence against their comrades as a result of torture, or fear of reprisals by agents of the former government.

During apartheid, many South Africans were exposed to political violence in their communities, at the hands of the security forces or as the result of conflict between different political factions in the community. The TRC termed those forms of violence which occurred outside the context of detention or confinement 'severe ill-treatment'. The most common forms of severe ill-treatment that were reported were arson (for example, homes or property being set on fire), being beaten, and being shot by security forces during mass protests.[10] At the TRC, severe ill-treatment was the category of violation most commonly reported by women, particularly those in the 37–48-year age group.[11] In the SASH survey, political violence that occurred outside the context of detention and torture was the most common form of political trauma reported by both men and women.[12]

Political violence in South Africa, whether it occurred in the context of detention or in the broader community, was often fatal. Nearly 10,000 politically motivated killings were reported to the TRC by surviving family members of the victims,[13] and these are likely to represent only a portion of politically motivated deaths during apartheid. The victims of these killings were predominantly young black men. These sudden, violent deaths left many more thousands of family members suffering from traumatic bereavement. In addition, many families endured the trauma of having a family member disappear without explanation or return, as the result of being abducted (and, according to later investigations by the TRC, subsequently killed) by state security forces. A project of the Centre for the Study of Violence and Reconciliation (CSVR) concerned with the TRC and its long-term impact has established a database to record such disappearances and has also documented some of the experiences of family members of the disappeared.[14]

The high rates of exposure to political violence in the South African population are an indication of the degree to which the struggle against apartheid was a mass, community-based, nationwide struggle that was not restricted to a small group of political activists or to particular regions of the country. While black male youth and children were often on the 'front lines' of this struggle, adult men and women were also targets of political violence perpetrated by the state. As a result, there are few, if any, segments of the current adult black South African population that have not been directly exposed to the political violence of the apartheid years.

Although the excesses of apartheid era violence are now in the past, contemporary South African society is not free of political violence. Some of this violence has its roots in the past. For example, there is still periodic conflict in KwaZulu-Natal between African National Congress (ANC) and Inkatha Freedom Party (IFP) office bearers and supporters. Other issues are more recent in origin. Conflict between citizens and the state has resulted in violence in certain instances, and worker and community protests have been harshly subdued on occasion, with reports of police personnel using rubber bullets and tear-gas to disperse protestors. The xenophobic attacks against people who have settled in South Africa from other countries that occurred nationwide during 2008 resulted in deaths and injuries, and in broad terms are a form of political violence, as many of these attacks were driven by perceived competition for jobs and resources.

Researchers at the CSVR have also pointed out that it is sometimes difficult to draw the line between political and criminal violence. For example, there is some evidence that alienated ex-liberation soldiers have become involved in violent crime,[15] and high levels of criminal activity in South Africa have their roots in the long political history of colonisation and oppression that has created major wealth disparities, high unemployment levels, and a fracturing of traditional family and community structures. We turn now to the prevalence of criminal violence in South Africa.

Criminal violence
In a 2007 review of violent crime in South Africa compared with elsewhere in the world, Altbeker concluded that 'South Africa ranks at the very top of the world's league tables for violent crime.'[16] This situation has most likely arisen as the result of a complex interplay of

factors that are unique to South Africa, which Altbeker and others[17] have discussed at length.

For several years since the late 1990s, South Africa has had one of the highest murder and armed robbery rates globally.[18] In a study of the global burden of disease, South Africa's homicide rate was more than five times the global average and 30 per cent higher than that of other countries in Sub-Saharan Africa.[19] In Canada, Australia and many western European countries, murder rates average less than two people per 100,000 in the population. In the United States, which is commonly criticised for its 'gun culture', there are approximately five murders per 100,000 people. In those economically developing countries for which some statistics are available (such as India, Chile and Nigeria), murder rates range from three to about twenty per 100,0000. However, in South Africa in 2006 the murder rate was forty-one people per 100 000, which translates into approximately fifty murders every day.[20] This in turn means that, each day, there are hundreds of South Africans who are deeply traumatised by learning of the violent death of a loved one.

In the SASH survey of adults in South Africa, 18 per cent of participants reported being a direct victim of a non-sexual violent crime.[21] However, men were at greater risk of criminal victimisation than women: 26 per cent of men reported exposure to criminal violence, compared with 12 per cent of women. Mortality surveys in South Africa have also found that young men are by far the most frequent victims of violent assault.[22] This is in line with research in other countries, such as the United States, Canada and Mexico, which have consistently found that men are most frequently the targets of violence outside the home, and particularly of attacks involving a weapon.[23] However, in South Africa a substantial portion of violence between men appears to occur outside of the context of traditional criminal activities such as committing a robbery. Given the high level of involvement of young South African men in gang activity,[24] it is likely that many violent assaults and homicides occur through inter-gang violence. In addition, there is evidence from mortality surveys to suggest that violence between South African males often happens in the context of entertainment and is related to high levels of alcohol consumption during recreational periods such as weekends and holidays.[25] As such, male-on-male violence in South Africa is not always criminal in nature (that is, perpetrated during the commission of a crime) but rather is an expression of normative notions of masculine behaviour that include the carrying of weapons, gang membership, risk-taking, defending one's honour, and excessive alcohol consumption.[26]

At the same time, there is also a high incidence of violence during the commission of more traditional criminal activities in South Africa. Robberies in South Africa are much more likely to involve the use of a weapon than robberies in other countries. Some surveys have found that as many as 80 per cent of serious robberies reported to the South African Police involve the use of a firearm, compared with less than 20 per cent in economically developed countries. Robberies also frequently involve the use of other weapons such as knives.[27] In addition to armed robberies that occur in the victim's home, in the street or on public transport, armed car hijackings and cash-in-transit heists are prominent forms of victimisation in South Africa. In the SASH study, participants living in urban areas were more likely to have experienced a violent crime than those living in less urbanised regions,[28] which is in keeping with the trends in other countries. Interestingly, while studies in the United States have found that members of minority ethnic groups in the population tend to be more exposed to criminal violence,[29] in the SASH study there were no significant differences across race and language groups in the percentage of South African adults who had experienced a violent crime outside the home.[30]

While the SASH study focused on adults, there is also evidence that South African youth are at high risk of being exposed to criminal violence. In a school survey of Grade 10 learners at both low and high socio-economic status schools in the Western Cape, almost a third reported that they had been robbed or mugged.[31] In a national youth victimisation survey of over 4,000 adolescents, 9 per cent had been robbed, 10 per cent reported a housebreaking at their home, and 10 per cent had experienced a car hijacking.[32] Overall, young people in South Africa are twice as likely as adults to be victims of at least one crime, with boys being more at risk of non-sexual crimes than girls.[33]

Gender-based violence

While South African men are most likely to be the victims of criminal violence, South African women and girls are at high risk of experiencing intimate partner abuse and sexual violence or coercion. The term 'gender-based violence' has several definitions (including emotional and economic abuse of women), but for our purposes here, it will be used to refer specifically to physical and sexual assaults against females by males. Gender-based violence includes physical and sexual assaults perpetrated by intimate partners (commonly termed domestic violence or intimate partner violence), as well as physical and sexual assaults by non-partners.

In South Africa and elsewhere, reliable statistics on the prevalence of gender-based violence are difficult to obtain because in many cases violence against women remains unreported. This occurs for many reasons, including women's emotional and economic dependency on the abuser, fear of further punishment by the abuser, lack of confidence in the police and fear of being further victimised by the criminal justice system, the absence of any nearby police stations, feelings of shame and self-blame, or an acceptance of the abuse as normal, deserved or a private matter that should not be disclosed.[34] Furthermore, police statistics tend to classify reported acts of gender-based violence under more general categories such as assault or attempted murder, which do not reflect the gender of the victim.[35] In South Africa, there is a substantial difference in the number of cases of sexual violence that are reported to the police and the number of cases that are reported by women participating in research studies (where women are usually able to remain anonymous and can avoid any negative consequences of reporting the abuse), with the number of reported cases being up to nine times higher in the latter.[36] So, while it is likely that community-based research studies may also under-represent rates of gender-based violence to some extent, they do seem to yield a more accurate picture than official police statistics.

In 1999, a review of research surveys of physical violence against women in close to fifty different countries (including economically developed and developing countries) indicated high but varying prevalence rates across countries, with between 10 and 50 per cent of women reporting that they had been physically abused by their partners.[37] In South Africa, the nationally representative SASH study conducted from 2002 found that 14 per cent of adult women reported having experienced physical abuse by an intimate partner.[38] Similarly, a 1998 nationally representative survey of health issues among nearly 12,000 South African women aged between fifteen and forty-nine years (the South African Demographic and Health Survey or SADHS) found that about 13 per cent had been physically abused by an intimate partner.[39] However, in the national SASH survey 28 per cent of men reported that they had physically abused an intimate partner,[40] suggesting that rates of intimate partner abuse may be much higher than female research participants admit.

There are significant regional variations in the reported prevalence of intimate partner abuse in South Africa. In the SADHS survey of women, the highest levels of intimate partner violence were reported in Gauteng (17.8 per cent) and the Western Cape (16.9 per cent).[41] A subsequent smaller survey, which focused specifically on gender-based violence in the three provinces of Mpumulanga, Eastern Cape and Northern Province (and was therefore named the Three Province Study) found much higher prevalence rates of intimate partner violence in these three provinces than had been found by the SADHS study, with substantially higher rates reported by women in Mpumulanga (28 per cent) and the Eastern Cape (27 per cent), compared with the Northern Province (19 per cent).[42] Some studies among specific communities in South Africa have found even higher levels of partner abuse. For example, 50 per cent of the women attending an antenatal clinic in Soweto reported that they had experienced intimate partner violence,[43] 80 per cent of a sample of women in rural communities in the southern Cape reported experiences of domestic violence,[44] and 42 per cent of male municipal workers in Cape Town[45] and about one third of a sample of young men from seventy villages in the rural Eastern Cape[46] reported that they had been physically abusive towards their female partners. It is also apparent that many South African women in abusive relationships experience a combination of different forms of abuse, including physical, sexual and emotional abuse.[47]

While available statistics do not necessarily indicate that rates of intimate partner violence are higher in South Africa than elsewhere, there is some evidence to suggest that rates of sexual violence are exceptionally high in South Africa compared with the rest of the world. In 1995, the Human Rights Watch report labelled South Africa as the rape capital of the world[48] and a 1999 comparison of South Africa with eighty-nine Interpol member states found that South Africa had the highest ratio of reported rape cases per 100,000 in the population.[49] While comparisons to other countries are somewhat limited by the fact that the legal definition of rape varies across different countries, it is clear that South African women are at enormously high risk of sexual victimisation.

The results of research surveys (which rely on subjective perceptions about whether one has been raped or sexually abused, rather than on legal definitions) confirm that rates of rape and other forms of sexual assault are high in South Africa, although not always higher than those reported in other countries. The SADHS study referred to earlier found that 7 per cent of the total sample of women had been forced to have sex against their will, and the Three Province Study reported similar prevalence rates of between 6 and 7 percent across the three provinces. These rates are higher than the rape rates reported in some national surveys in other countries, such as Mexico (3.9 per cent), Chile (3.8 per cent) and Australia (5.4 per cent),[50] but lower than those reported in the United States (9.2 per cent) and Canada (15.5 per cent).[51] Compared with the SADHS study, the more recent SASH study in South Africa found a much lower reported rate of rape (3.7 per cent) among women,[52] as well as a lower rate of sexual molestation (2.1 per cent) compared with countries such as the United States (12.3 per cent), Mexico (10.5 per cent) and Australia (10.2 per cent).[53] While this finding may possibly reflect a downward trend in the national prevalence of rape in South Africa since the SADHS study was conducted, the different rates of reported sexual violence and coercion are more likely due to methodological differences across the studies, such as sampling differences (for example, the SADHS study included women from the age of fifteen years old, while the SASH study included women from the age of eighteen), the use of different measuring instruments, different forms of training provided to interviewers, and differences arising from the translation of questions about sexual assault into a number of South African languages.

Some studies indicate that women in specific communities in South Africa are at a much higher risk of sexual violence than is reflected in the national average that has been reported in the different surveys in South Africa. For example, the study of women attending an antenatal clinic in Soweto referred to earlier, found that 20 per cent reported experiencing sexual violence by an intimate partner,[54] and it appears that younger South African women are at much higher risk of being raped than older women.[55]

Although reliable statistics for violence against children are particularly difficult to establish, South Africa does appear to have a disturbingly high rate of childhood sexual abuse. In South Africa in 2004 more than 40 per cent of all rapes reported to the police, and nearly half of indecent assaults, were perpetrated against children. In numbers this amounted to almost 25,000 children, and since only about one in twenty cases of child sexual abuse are reported, it is likely that between 400,000 and 500,000 children are raped in South Africa every year.[56] Furthermore, sexual abuse of children is one of the few forms of violence in South Africa that is actually increasing over time. This is contrary to the trend in the United States, which has seen a decline in rates of child sexual victimisation since the early 1990s.[57]

Some prevalence studies conducted with South African adult women have asked retrospectively about their experiences of sexual abuse in childhood. The SADHS study found that 1.6 per cent of women reported having been forced to have sex against their will before the age of fifteen,[58] while the Three Province Study similarly found that 1.2 per cent had been raped, and 3.3 per cent had experienced unwanted sexual contact, before the age of fifteen years.[59] However, the average rate of childhood sexual victimisation reported in very large surveys can obscure the much higher risk to some girls as opposed to others. For example, the survey of three secondary schools in the Western Cape region, referred to previously in this chapter, reported that 17 per cent of female adolescents had experienced a sexual assault,[60] while a survey of female secondary school students in the Northern Province found that over 50 per cent had experienced unwanted sexual contact.[61] Being forced to have sex against their will by a dating partner was reported by 28 per cent of a sample of female school students in the Transkei[62] and by 28 per cent of a random sample of young women from Umlazi, Khayelitsha and Soweto.[63] Studies of female university students have reported that between 23 and 53 per cent had experienced some form of unwanted sexual touching (including rape) in childhood.[64] These rates are higher than those found in community-based studies with adult women in the United States where, on average, about 20 per cent of participants have reported being sexually abused in childhood.[65] Most rapes of young girls in South Africa are perpetrated by men known to the victim, including relatives, neighbours and school teachers,[66] and since most sexual violence is not reported to the police, many young rape survivors face the trauma of ongoing daily contact with the rapist.

In keeping with international findings, South African women are not the only victims of sexual violence and coercion. In the national SASH study, 0.3 per cent of men reported that they had been raped while 1 per cent reported experiencing other forms of sexual coercion.[67] Studies of male secondary school and university students have reported that between 9 and 56 per cent have experienced unwanted sexual contact in childhood,[68] and another study found that, between 2001 and 2003, 131 sexually abused boys presented to a medico-legal centre in KwaZulu-Natal.[69] In an epidemiological study conducted in three districts of the Eastern Cape and KwaZulu-Natal, 4.6 per cent of men reported being raped in the past year.[70]

The reported rates of sexual violence in all the research studies discussed above must be viewed as an under-representation of the true state of affairs, since incidents of sexual coercion (particularly in marital, dating and familial relationships) are likely to be under-reported.[71] Although we must rely on research data as a guideline, it is likely that the true prevalence of sexual violence and coercion experienced by South Africans is unfortunately far higher than even our best data suggests. For example, in the epidemiological study of men in the Eastern Cape and KwaZulu-Natal, 27.6 per cent of the participants admitted to having raped at least one person.[72] As with intimate partner abuse, this suggests that the true prevalence of rape in South Africa may be a good deal higher than is revealed by studies that have asked women whether they have been raped.

In addition, statistics on the prevalence of gender-based violence do not necessarily reflect the severity of violence against women in South Africa. The degree of violence associated with domestic abuse and sexual assaults in South Africa appears to be particularly extreme. With regard to intimate partner violence, South African women are killed by their male partners six times more often than the international average.[73] For sexual assaults, one regional study found that rapes in the Western Cape are twelve times more likely to be fatal than sexual assaults in the United States,[74] while there is also evidence to suggest that the national prevalence of rape homicides in South Africa is higher than that of *all* female homicides in the United States.[75] Furthermore, the emotional and physical trauma of rape in South Africa is often exacerbated by assaults from more than one rapist, with gang rape being reported by a quarter to one-third of all South African rape survivors who presented to medico-legal clinics in Johannesburg[76] and by a third of all participants in a study of 250 rape survivors from three provinces.[77]

Childhood physical abuse

The prevalence of physical abuse of children by a family member is extremely difficult to estimate reliably – once again, police statistics reflect only the reported cases, which represent a very small minority of all incidents, and for a number of reasons it is extremely difficult to interview children directly about their experiences of physical abuse. One way to estimate rates of childhood physical abuse is to ask adults whether they were abused in childhood. While this only provides a picture of the prevalence of childhood physical abuse in the past, rather than the present, it does give an indication of the number of South Africans who may be living with the trauma of an abusive childhood. In the SASH survey of South African adults, 12 per cent of participants reported that they had experienced physical abuse by a caregiver in childhood.[78] This is several times higher than the rates found in a national survey in the United States.[79] With regard to who is most at risk of childhood physical abuse by a family member, some United States studies indicate that males are more vulnerable than females, while others report that both genders are equally at risk across all ages.[80] In the SASH survey there was little difference in the rate of childhood physical abuse reported by males and females,[81] but reviews of local hospital records suggest that the majority of children injured by domestic physical abuse are boys under the age of five years.[82]

Non-Intentional Injury

Although it is difficult to obtain reliable and systematic data about the prevalence of accidental injury, information from mortality studies (which track the causes of fatal injuries in the population) suggests that South Africa has a high rate of injuries due to accidental causes. For example, like many other countries in Sub-Saharan Africa, South Africa has a death rate from unintentional injuries that is about 30 per cent higher than the global average, with our most common forms of accidental injury being road traffic injuries and burn injuries.[83]

Road traffic injuries

South Africa's death rate from traffic accidents (forty-three per 100,000 people in the population) is double the global average.[84] Approximately one quarter of all injury-related deaths in South Africa occur as the result of road traffic accidents. Injuries to pedestrians, rather than to vehicle passengers, are the most common form of traffic-related injury in South Africa, accounting for about 40 per cent of all traffic-related deaths.[85] With regard to non-fatal traffic injuries, in 2005, it was estimated that about one hundred South Africans were seriously injured in road traffic accidents every day, and twenty of these were permanently disabled.[86] However, a traffic accident does not have to result in an injury to be psychologically traumatic: as we shall see in the next chapter, any event that is experienced as being life-threatening can result in post-traumatic stress symptoms. In the SASH survey, 12.2 per cent of participants reported that they had been involved in a life-threatening car accident.[87]

Those most at risk of being injured in a traffic accident are males from socio-economically disadvantaged communities, who make up the majority of pedestrians in South Africa. Indeed, road traffic collisions were ranked as the fourth leading cause of death among South African males in 2000.[88] However, the number of deaths due to road traffic accidents is much higher for both sexes in South Africa compared with many other countries.[89]

Burn injuries

The main victims of accidental burn injuries in South Africa are children. Burn injuries are a leading cause of injury, disability and non-natural death among South African children, especially those between the ages of one and five years old.[90] One study conducted in the Western Cape found that six children per every 10,000 in the population are seriously burned, and noted that the risk of a burn injury is heightened by conditions of poverty, which are characterised by overcrowding, the use of a single room for cooking, washing and living, and the use of non-electrical sources of energy like paraffin and candles.[91] South African children living in poor households are therefore most likely to be the victims of a burn injury.

Among children, it is infants and toddlers who are most at risk of being burnt, and scalding by boiling water is the most common form of burn injury in this age group. While infant boys are generally more likely than infant girls to sustain a scalding injury, in the toddler age range females appear to be more vulnerable. Older children, and again females in particular, are most likely to sustain flame burns – because they are more mobile and independent than infants. Due to gender role expectations girl children are more exposed to activities such as cooking and the lighting of fires.[92]

Indirect Traumatisation

Research in countries such as the United States and Canada has established that one does not need to be a direct victim of a trauma in order to develop posttraumatic symptoms.[93] Even being indirectly exposed to a situation where someone else's physical safety is under threat can result in a similar response to that which is common after being directly traumatised.[94] Indirect forms of traumatisation include witnessing violence or injury to another person (for example, an act of criminal violence, a serious traffic accident or a burn injury to a child), as well as hearing about a trauma that occurred to someone close, such as a family member or close friend. A trauma to a close other is

23

particularly likely to cause distress and posttraumatic symptoms if the trauma is fatal, resulting in a traumatic bereavement.[95]

Indirect forms of trauma exposure are very common in South African society. In the SASH study, 28 per cent of the sample reported that they had witnessed a traumatic event, such as someone being injured or killed.[96] This is comparable to rates of witnessing trauma that have been found in other countries. Also consistent with findings in other countries, such as the United States, Canada, Australia and Mexico,[97] South African men were more likely than women to report witnessing a traumatic event, especially violence. It is possible that men are more likely than women to witness violent incidents because, due to traditional gender-role expectations, they spend more time in the public sphere outside the home.

In the SASH survey, hearing about a trauma to a close other was more common than witnessing a trauma, with 43 per cent of the sample reporting such an experience. In most cases, the trauma involved the unexpected death of a loved one, and women were more likely to have experienced a sudden bereavement than men.[98] This is not surprising since, as we have seen throughout this chapter, South African males have been the predominant victims of political violence, criminal violence and accidental injuries, leaving many South African women to mourn the sudden and traumatic loss of their partners, fathers, brothers and sons.

Multiple Traumatisation

As can be seen from the information presented in this chapter so far, there are many different forms of trauma that affect the South African population, including trauma in the home and in the broader community, and encompassing both direct and indirect forms of traumatisation. It is therefore to be expected that many South Africans have survived not just one traumatic experience in their lifetime, but several. Indeed, the SASH survey found that 56 per cent of respondents had experienced more than one trauma, and 16 per cent had experienced as many as four or five traumas.[99]

Multiple traumatisation can occur over a long period of time and presents the person with ongoing challenges to their attempts to recover and move forward with their life goals. For example, a 23-year-old woman living in Cape Town was admitted to a psychiatric hospital after being raped by a friend of her boyfriend. When the clinician interviewed her, it emerged that she had been sexually abused by her mother's brother for several years as a child. Then, when she was eighteen years old, she was gang-raped while walking home from the bus-stop after work. She had previously told no one about these experiences, but after the latest rape she felt too unsafe to leave her house at all, believed that life held no future for her, and had completely withdrawn from her work and social life. In another example of multiple traumatisation, a 53-year-old man was referred to counselling at a trauma clinic after being assaulted and robbed by gang members with knives at a taxi rank one evening. It emerged that in his twenties he had been detained and tortured by security police over a period of three months because of his political activities, and as a result of his torture-related injuries he experienced severe back pain that limited his capacity to sustain employment. Furthermore, he had experienced a traumatic bereavement when his son died three years before in a car accident. Thus it is apparent that those who are multiply traumatised may experience separate incidences of both related and unrelated kinds of traumatic events. In both instances the impact of later traumas is likely to be compounded by prior exposure as will be discussed in more detail in subsequent chapters.

Despite the popular belief that South Africans are exposed to more trauma than citizens in other countries, experiences of multiple traumatisation have been reported across many different countries. Although it is difficult to make direct comparisons with the SASH survey due to the use of different instruments to measure trauma exposure across different studies, similar or even higher rates of multiple trauma exposure have been reported in national surveys in the United States, Canada and Mexico.[100] Consistent across all these studies, including the SASH survey, is the finding that men are at significantly higher risk than women of being exposed to multiple traumas.

Conclusion
This chapter has focused on patterns of direct and indirect exposure to some of the most common forms of intentional violence and non-

intentional injury in South Africa. There are, of course, other forms of traumatisation that are common among the South African population. This includes receiving a diagnosis of a life-threatening illness such as HIV/AIDS,[101] and injuries that are sustained as a result of work-related accidents (particularly in the mining sector).[102] Furthermore, natural disasters such as floods, or the tornado that left many people homeless in Cape Town in 1999, and the subsequent dislocation caused by these events, are also traumatic. It is often the poor and marginalised who are most affected by natural disasters. For example, those most likely to be living below flood-lines and therefore most vulnerable to risk in heavy storms are people living in informal housing. Finally, it is important to note that being the perpetrator of violence or injury, whether accidental or intentional, can also be experienced as traumatic.[103]

Research has not consistently supported the popular notion that South Africans, as a whole, are exposed to more trauma than people living in other countries, but there is an accumulation of disturbing evidence that interpersonal violence in South Africa takes a more severe and lethal form than the international norm. Almost half of all South African deaths due to injury are the result of interpersonal violence, which is four-and-a-half times the rate of violence-related deaths internationally.[104] Violence between young men (often in the context of gang activity or alcohol-related entertainment), and sexual and physical violence towards women and children all take a particularly brutal form compared with such interpersonal violence in many other countries. As such, the stereotype of South Africa as a particularly dangerous society does appear to be supported by systematic evidence. However, the greatest burden of trauma exposure falls upon South Africans who have historically been the victims of political oppression (under the recent apartheid system but also within the broader historical context of colonisation), many of whom still continue to live in conditions of poverty and disempowerment. In this sense, trauma exposure in post-apartheid South Africa remains a deeply political issue, rooted in historical dynamics of power and inequality.

Because the majority of South Africans have experienced at least one trauma, and many have suffered multiple traumatic experiences, it appears that trauma is not an extraordinary or aberrant event in our

26

society, but rather a commonplace one. This raises some important questions. Just because trauma is common, does this normalise it? Do people living in conditions of chronic violence and traumatisation eventually become desensitised to trauma and find functional ways to cope and adapt, or are they in fact more at risk for psychiatric disorders and other problems in living? Do South Africans who live with daily violence construct traumatised identities or subjectivities for themselves (that is, do they think about themselves as being 'traumatised' or suffering from 'trauma'), in the absence of trauma-free norms against which to measure their experience? Local research has begun to tackle some of these complex questions, although there is still much that remains to be understood about how South Africans adapt to conditions of multiple and continuous exposure to potentially traumatic events, and how historical oppression as well as ongoing conditions of poverty and inequality contribute to the meaning and impact of trauma exposure across different South African communities. The next two chapters will examine what we currently know about the psychological impact of trauma exposure, from both local and international research.

Chapter 3

POSTTRAUMATIC STRESS DISORDER AND OTHER TRAUMA SYNDROMES

In general, human beings have a remarkable capacity to adapt to extreme stress from the environment. The majority of survivors of potentially traumatic events experience a brief period of disequilibrium, but do not develop lasting difficulties. However, a substantial minority go on to experience severe and ongoing symptoms that cause much distress and substantially restrict their ability to function in the world. When trauma responses reach this level, they may be classified as a psychiatric disorder. Posttraumatic Stress Disorder (PTSD)[1] is the most widely publicised trauma-related psychiatric disorder and it will therefore be a major focus of this chapter, but there are several others that are also commonly associated with traumatic events. In addition, researchers have recently attempted to describe the psychological and psychiatric effects of prolonged abuse at the hands of another person, and the ways in which these differ from the effects of single traumas. Despite significant advances in our understanding of trauma-related syndromes, in this chapter we will also see that relatively little is known about the effects of exposure to continuous community violence, a context that many South Africans currently live in. Finally, this chapter will review existing South African research on the psychiatric impact of trauma exposure in South Africa, and consider some of the gaps in our local knowledge that require further attention.

Posttraumatic Stress Disorder

Normal trauma reactions versus PTSD

After a traumatic event, most people will experience some degree of distress as they try to adapt to what has happened. Common reactions include feelings of anxiety and mild depression, having distressing thoughts and memories of the traumatic event, difficulty sleeping, and feeling hyper-alert to any signs of danger. In order to manage these symptoms, many trauma survivors may wish to avoid talking about what happened, may withdraw from contact with other people, and may feel emotionally numb when they think about the trauma.[2] These reactions can last for a few days, weeks or even months after the traumatic event and then gradually fade, without severely impacting on the survivor's ability to continue with their normal daily functioning.

However, for some trauma survivors the above symptoms do not gradually diminish over time and continue to create substantial impairment in their work and social roles. Posttraumatic Stress Disorder is a psychiatric diagnosis that has been developed to describe such a response to trauma. PTSD was first introduced as a psychiatric disorder in 1980, but since then the diagnostic criteria for PTSD have been further refined through systematic clinical research, largely based in North America. The current diagnostic criteria for PTSD are presented in Box 3.1.

The first requirement for the PTSD diagnosis is that the person must have experienced a traumatic event (either as a direct victim or as a witness) that involved some form of physical threat. Historically, the term 'trauma' has been used to refer to a wide variety of experiences, including emotionally stressful ones. For example, in the psychoanalytic tradition, the term 'trauma' is often used to refer to emotionally damaging life experiences, such as having extremely critical or emotionally unresponsive caregivers – in this sense, trauma is an emotional injury, rather than a physical one. However, research has shown that the specific syndrome of PTSD is typically linked to

Box 3.1 DSM-IV-TR Diagnostic Criteria for PTSD

A. The person has been exposed to a traumatic event in which both of the following were present:
   (1) the person experienced, witnessed, or was confronted with an event or events that involved actual or threatened death or serious injury, or threat to the physical integrity of self or others
   (2) the person's response involved intense fear, helplessness, or horror

B. The traumatic event is persistently re-experienced in one (or more) of the following ways:
   (1) recurrent and intrusive distressing recollections of the event, including images, thoughts or perceptions
   (2) recurrent distressing dreams of the event
   (3) acting or feeling as if the traumatic event were recurring (includes a sense of reliving the experience, illusions, hallucinations, and dissociative flashback episodes)
   (4) intense psychological distress at exposure to internal or external cues that symbolise or resemble an aspect of the traumatic event
   (5) physiological reactivity on exposure to internal or external cues that symbolise or resemble an aspect of the traumatic event

C. Persistent avoidance of stimuli associated with the trauma and numbing of general responsiveness (not present before the trauma), as indicated by three (or more) of the following:
   (1) efforts to avoid thoughts, feelings, or conversations associated with the trauma
   (2) efforts to avoid activities, places, or people that arouse recollections of the trauma
   (3) inability to recall an important aspect of the trauma
   (4) markedly diminished interest or participation in significant activities
   (5) feelings of detachment or estrangement from others
   (6) restricted range of affect (for example, unable to have loving feelings)
   (7) sense of a foreshortened future (for example, does not expect to have a career, marriage, children, or a normal life span)

D. Persistent symptoms of increased arousal (not present before the trauma), as indicated by two (or more) of the following:
   (1) difficulty falling or staying asleep
   (2) irritability or outbursts of anger
   (3) difficulty concentrating
   (4) hypervigilance
   (5) exaggerated startle response

E. Duration of the disturbance (symptoms in Criteria B, C, and D) is more than 1 month

F. The disturbance causes clinically significant distress or impairment in social, occupational, or other important areas of functioning

Source: American Psychiatric Association, 2000.

physically threatening experiences, rather than emotionally damaging experiences that lack any perceived physical threat.[3] This is why the first diagnostic requirement for PTSD specifies that the person must have experienced an event perceived to be physically threatening. However, this criterion acknowledges that many people can develop PTSD from witnessing traumatic events, even if they have not been directly traumatised.

The diagnosis of PTSD also currently requires that the physically threatening event must have elicited a reaction of intense fear, helplessness or horror. This acknowledges that the person's subjective response to the event (how frightened they felt) is as important as the objective degree of physical threat involved. For example, one person may be mugged by an assailant who brandishes a firearm, and another by an unarmed assailant who verbally threatens to harm the person, but the second crime victim may feel subjectively more frightened and helpless than the first. The assumption behind this diagnostic requirement is that it is the subjective feeling of 'helpless terror'[4] during the trauma that is implicated in the development of PTSD. However, this criterion has been somewhat controversial, since there is not strong evidence to show that a fearful response during a traumatic event predicts the development of PTSD.[5]

In addition to specifying the type of traumatic experience that qualifies a person to be considered for the diagnosis, there are three clusters of symptoms for PTSD. The first symptom cluster includes different forms of re-experiencing the trauma in a manner that the trauma survivor is unable to voluntarily control. For example, the survivor may find that throughout the day images and thoughts about the trauma continually intrude into their consciousness, despite their best efforts to block these out. At night, this intrusion may occur in the form of nightmares about the trauma. In addition, whenever the person encounters something that reminds them of the trauma (known as a traumatic 'trigger') they feel intense distress and fear, and experience physical symptoms associated with the body's natural response to danger (known as the 'fight, flight or freeze' response), including increased heart rate, muscle tension and sweating.[6] Finally, the survivor may experience flashbacks about the trauma, especially when they encounter a traumatic reminder or trigger. Flashbacks differ from normal memories as they involve intense sensory re-experiencing of the trauma (smelling the same smells, hearing the same sounds, feeling the same sensations on the skin), rather than just an image or thought about the event. Through all these symptoms, the survivor finds themselves perpetually stuck in the moment of the trauma. At least one form of re-experiencing the trauma must be present in order to qualify for a possible diagnosis of PTSD.

The second symptom cluster of PTSD involves avoidance symptoms. In an attempt to manage the highly distressing re-experiencing symptoms described above, the trauma survivor may attempt to avoid any reminders of the trauma. For example, the person may make a conscious effort to avoid places or situations that are associated with the trauma. A hijack victim may try to avoid having to drive anywhere alone (see the case study in Box 3.2), a child who has been mugged outside his school may refuse to go back to school afterwards, and a woman who has been raped while walking to her bus stop may feel unable to walk that route again or to use any form of public transport. This avoidance may not be restricted to the trauma-specific situation, but may also generalise to the point where the person avoids leaving their home at all, or only goes out when absolutely necessary, and this may substantially restrict their participation in their usual activities.

Trauma survivors also often wish to avoid talking to others about the trauma, as this makes them feel anxious and distressed all over again. For many survivors, talking about or remembering the trauma feels as dangerous as actually experiencing it. This may be hard for family and friends to understand, as there is a popular notion that trauma survivors should talk about what happened in order to feel better. Survivors may also find that they attempt not to think about the trauma at all, forcing themselves to think about something else if a thought about the trauma enters their mind. Usually these attempts at mental avoidance are only partially successful, and intrusive thoughts and images repeatedly push their way into consciousness. In addition, the survivor may try to avoid the distressing feelings associated with the trauma by numbing themselves emotionally, resulting in feeling cut-off or emotionally detached much of the time. At least three of the avoidance symptoms listed in Box 3.1 must be present in order to consider a possible diagnosis of PTSD.

The final symptom cluster of PTSD is an increased level of physical arousal (known as hyperarousal) compared with before the trauma. This physical arousal entails an ongoing state of the body's 'fight, flight or freeze' response, and involves difficulty sleeping, difficulty concentrating on daily activities, being constantly on the look out for signs of threat and danger (known as hypervigilance), being startled very easily at loud noises or sudden movements, and becoming easily irritable or angry in response to minor frustrations or perceived hostility from others. At least two of these symptoms must be present in order for the survivor to qualify for a possible diagnosis of PTSD.

As noted earlier, it is normal to experience many of these symptoms for a while after the trauma, and their presence alone is not sufficient to diagnose PTSD. To meet the diagnosis, the re-experiencing, avoidance and hyperarousal symptoms must be present for at least one month after the trauma *and* they must cause the person extreme distress or interfere significantly with their ability to function at work or in their social roles. A careful assessment by a psychologist or psychiatrist is necessary in order to establish whether the full criteria for PTSD are met.

The course of PTSD varies over time. Research indicates that about half of the people who develop PTSD will recover within three months (this is called Acute PTSD). For others, the symptoms will come and go for months or years after the trauma (Chronic PTSD), and still others may only develop PTSD six months or more after the actual trauma (Delayed PTSD).[7] A diagnosis that is closely related to PTSD is Acute Stress Disorder or ASD. This diagnosis can be made if symptoms of PTSD are present for less than one month and there are also prominent features of *dissociation*, which may occur either during the traumatic event or afterwards.[8] Dissociation includes a sense of emotional numbing or detachment, a reduced awareness of one's surroundings (for example, feeling as if one is in a daze), amnesia for certain aspects of the trauma, feeling detached from one's body or feeling that the world is unreal or dreamlike. While many trauma survivors may experience some symptoms of dissociation during or immediately after the trauma, the diagnosis of ASD is only made if these symptoms cause significant distress or create a serious impairment in the survivor's ability to function after the trauma. If the symptoms of ASD last longer than one month, the diagnosis may be changed to PTSD if the full diagnostic criteria for PTSD are met.

Box 3.2 Case study of PTSD

Five months ago, Thandi was hijacked in her driveway after coming home from a night class at the local Technikon. The hijackers were three men, each of whom carried a gun. One of them held a gun to her head during the hijacking. Her husband was not at home at the time, but her neighbours heard her screaming for help after the hijackers had fled with her car, and they called the police. Thandi's car was later found abandoned several blocks away.

Since the hijacking, Thandi has been experiencing the following symptoms. Each evening, as soon as it starts to get dark, she begins to feel highly anxious and fearful. She refuses to drive anywhere at night, even with somebody else, and this has meant that she has had to stop attending night classes. She is extremely hypervigilant when coming home, often driving past her driveway three or four times to make sure that no attackers are lurking there before she is willing to pull in and park at her home.

Several times a day she has flashbacks of the hijacking, in which she can hear the sounds of the hijackers shouting and of car doors slamming, smell the scent of cigarettes on the breath of the hijacker who was holding a gun to her head, and feel the cold sensation of the gun at her temple. The flashbacks are often brought on when she hears the sound of men shouting or of car doors slamming, or when she smells cigarettes on someone's breath. During the flashbacks, her heart thumps wildly, she shakes, and she feels like she cannot breathe. She also has nightmares in which the hijacking is replayed. She wakes up and feels so anxious that she cannot fall asleep again, and lies awake in a tense state, listening out for any noises which might indicate that an intruder is on the property.

At work, she is unable to concentrate and often finds her attention drifting for long periods of time. She has also become very irritable with her work colleagues and they have taken to avoiding her unless they absolutely have to speak to her.

Thandi's husband has tried to talk with her about how she's feeling, but Thandi insists that she just wants to 'forget about what happened and move on – there's no point dwelling on it'. She becomes angry when friends tell her to 'talk about what happened – you'll feel better', and has started to avoid social arrangements.

Explanations for PTSD

Research outside of South Africa has consistently found that PTSD affects only a minority of trauma survivors. Although estimates vary across studies, depending on the kind of methodology that was used, it is evident that generally not more than 25 per cent of trauma survivors develop PTSD.[9] Several explanations have been offered to account for the development of PTSD in some trauma survivors but not others.

As suggested by PTSD symptoms such as flashbacks and intrusive images, traumatic memories have a very distinct quality compared with normal memories. There are several theories about why the traumatic memories that characterise PTSD are re-experienced in such an intrusive, vivid and uncontrollable way by some trauma survivors, compared with memories for non-traumatic events. For example, early psychoanalytic theorists proposed that the re-experiencing symptoms that often follow after a trauma are a form of repetition compulsion, whereby the mind unconsciously attempts to achieve psychological mastery over the traumatic event by replaying it repeatedly.[10] This attempt at mastery is part of the psyche's natural attempt to adapt to, and heal from, an intensely distressing experience. In the case of PTSD, however, this mechanism does not fade over time as the person adapts to what has happened, but rather continues to operate.

Other theorists have drawn on the concept of 'schemas' to explain the re-experiencing symptoms of PTSD. A schema is an internal cognitive structure or framework that organises and interprets information from our environment. Our existing schemas, which have developed from all our previous experience, provide a model of the world that guides our behaviour.[11] Schemas evolve through the dual processes of assimilation and accommodation. In the former, experiences that are familiar to the person's working model of the world are categorised and incorporated into their existing schemas, thereby strengthening these; in the latter, schemas are modified in order to account for novel experiences that cannot be categorised into existing schemas. Trauma theorists have argued that, for some trauma survivors, the traumatic experience may be too alien and too discrepant with previous experience to be either assimilated or accommodated into their existing schemas, resulting in the memory remaining disorganised.[12] When an experience defies cognitive categorisation, its memory may be incorporated as a purely sensory experience (sights, sounds, smells, bodily sensations and tastes), rather than as a narratively organised memory, that is, a memory with a coherent story to accompany it.[13] We will return to this notion of schemas in the next chapter, when we explore the ways in which people try to make meaning from traumatic experiences.

These cognitive theories are supported by evidence from brain imaging studies, which suggest that during a traumatic experience, extremely high levels of emotional arousal may prevent incoming information from being properly evaluated and categorised by a part of the brain known as the hippocampus.[14] Unlike other memories, traumatic memories may therefore not always be stored in the brain as a unified, integrated whole, but rather as sensory fragments.

But why do these unconscious, cognitive and neurobiological mechanisms become chronically disrupted for some trauma survivors, resulting in PTSD symptoms, while other trauma survivors develop only transitory symptoms? A number of factors have been identified that may contribute to the risk for developing PTSD. These factors are both biological and environmental.

Certain types of trauma appear to be more likely to produce PTSD than others. Studies in many different countries have consistently found that experiencing a violent assault is much more likely to result in PTSD than experiencing a traumatic accident or natural disaster. Furthermore, of all the different types of assaultive violence, sexual assault carries the highest risk of PTSD, for both men and women.[15] The SASH survey in South Africa similarly found that, for women, rape is far more likely to result in PTSD compared with other kinds of assault (for example, criminal violence or domestic abuse), although torture was the strongest predictor of PTSD for men.[16] Interestingly, despite the consistent finding that rape creates an exceptionally high risk for PTSD, there is almost no research that has tried to establish why this is so. Speculatively, this may be due to the intensely intrusive physical nature of the act of rape, or to environmental factors such as the lack of social support that rape survivors often encounter in their communities and from the medical or justice systems. How precisely these or other factors may increase the rape survivor's vulnerability to developing PTSD is still unclear – but clearly a matter requiring urgent attention in the South African context.

The female gender also appears to create a substantially higher risk for developing PTSD after a trauma. A number of studies in countries such as the United States, Canada, Mexico and Chile have indicated that women are at least twice as likely as men to develop PTSD after a trauma.[17] This holds true even when one takes into account that men and women tend to experience different kinds of trauma – in other words, this difference cannot be explained by the fact that women may experience more of the kinds of traumas that are likely to produce PTSD, such as sexual assault.[18] It remains unclear whether the higher risk for developing PTSD among women is due to biological factors (such as hormonal differences between men and women), differing environmental experiences (women are still generally more economically, educationally and politically disempowered than men, which may decrease their capacity to cope after trauma), different ways of coping with stress (for example, due to sex-role stereotypes, women may be more likely than men to acknowledge feeling fearful and avoidant of frightening situations, and more likely to seek help for these symptoms, so may be diagnosed with PTSD more often than men), or some combination of these factors.[19] Interestingly, however, both the SASH survey in South Africa[20] and an Australian survey[21] found no significant difference between men and women in rates of PTSD, suggesting that female gender may not necessarily pose a risk factor for PTSD in all societies.

It has also been established that the brain structure and functioning of trauma survivors who develop PTSD differ from those who do not develop PTSD. Firstly, brain imaging studies show that trauma survivors with PTSD have a significantly smaller hippocampus (an area of the brain which, as we have seen, plays a critical role in the categorisation and storage of incoming stimuli in memory) and an excessively activated amygdala (an area of the brain that is involved in evaluating the emotional significance of incoming stimuli).[22] People who develop PTSD after a trauma also appear to have a different type of neurochemical response to the trauma than those trauma survivors who do not develop PTSD. For example, the receptors in the brain for the stress hormone, cortisol, appear to be more sensitive in people who develop PTSD after a trauma, compared with those who do not, possibly making them intensely sensitive and hyper-responsive to external events.[23] This suggests that the neurobiology of PTSD is qualitatively different from the neurobiology of the normal stress response – that is, PTSD does not appear to be simply an extreme version of the normal stress response.

There has been some debate about whether these neurobiological features are inherited vulnerabilities that pre-date the trauma exposure, or whether they develop after the trauma as a result of the long-term impact of the extremely high stress levels that characterise PTSD. Studies comparing PTSD among fraternal and identical twins who have both survived trauma indicate that as much as 30 per cent of some PTSD symptoms may have a genetic basis.[24] Neuro-imaging evidence from studies where one twin has been exposed to trauma and has PTSD and the other twin has not been exposed to trauma indicates that a smaller hippocampus is a familial vulnerability that creates a greater risk for developing PTSD after experiencing a trauma.[25] Some people may therefore be physiologically more vulnerable to developing PTSD.

Research has shown that people with early childhood histories of trauma, and those with prior histories of mental illness or psychological difficulties, are more vulnerable to developing PTSD after experiencing a trauma later on in life.[26] These past experiences may create a vulnerability that causes the normal state of distress after a trauma to progress to more severe and lasting symptoms. However, the mechanism whereby prior psychological difficulties or previous traumas increase one's risk of PTSD are still unclear. In addition to past adversities, it is also apparent that current life stress places trauma survivors at greater risk of PTSD,[27] a noteworthy finding given the multiple life stressors experienced by South Africans living in conditions of poverty.

Finally, it appears that a lack of available support networks and a perceived negative response from others in the days and weeks following a trauma may increase the risk of developing PTSD.[28] While we know that there is a relationship between PTSD and poor social support, it is still unclear whether a lack of social support influences the development of PTSD, or whether PTSD symptoms (such as a wish to avoid speaking about the trauma) restrict the seeking of social support. More research on the precise relationship between social support and PTSD is therefore needed.[29]

Although much is known about the factors that create a risk or vulnerability for PTSD, less is known about the factors that protect against PTSD. This may be due to a bias in trauma research towards focusing on those trauma survivors who have developed PTSD rather than on those who have not. Research with people who recover from trauma may yield important information about the reasons for their recovery. At present there is some evidence to suggest that, while a lack of social support may increase risk for PTSD, good social support may be a strong protective factor. Some studies have shown that people who are able to talk to supportive friends and family about their memories of the traumatic event and their feelings of distress and anxiety appear to be less likely to develop ongoing PTSD symptoms than those who do not have a support network.[30] A South African study into the experiences of over a hundred victims of pre-election political violence on the East Rand found evidence confirming the centrality of social support in minimising symptom development.[31]

It is possible that social support is protective because it provides a means for the trauma survivor to cognitively process their memory of the event and the meaning that they assign to the event.[32] However, the role of social support as a protective factor is complex. Even people who receive a great deal of support after a trauma may go on to develop PTSD, suggesting that social support is only one of many factors that determine the long-term outcome of a trauma experience. Further, many traumatised people do not feel able to use their emotional support networks even when these are available, due to the need to avoid talking about the trauma or a fear that others will judge or blame them for responding inadequately during the trauma.[33]

There has also been some research into personality features that may counteract the impact of traumatic events. These include an internal or external locus of control (that is, a sense that control over one's life comes from within or outside of oneself, respectively),[34] hardiness (or resilience to stress)[35] and sense of coherence (that is, having a sense that life is meaningful, predictable and manageable).[36] Research into such personality features and coping styles has been extended from the general stress field into the traumatic stress field with some indications that these dimensions may assist in preventing trauma symptoms in specific populations. However, research into these and other possible protective factors in the context of trauma is ongoing. The possibility of finding strength and positive psychological growth through traumatic experiences will be discussed in more detail in the next chapter.

Many people with PTSD tend to blame themselves for being 'ill', and feel that their symptoms are a sign of personal weakness and incompetence.[37] However, given all the above evidence, it is likely that whether or not a trauma survivor develops PTSD is dependent upon a complex combination of different factors that we are only just beginning to understand. These include factors that pre-date the trauma (such as gender, genetic vulnerability, personality features and our cognitive schemas about the world), factors inherent in the trauma itself (such as the type of traumatic event) and post-trauma variables (such as social support and additional life stress). Overall, it appears that factors operating during and after the trauma are more likely to result in PTSD than pre-existing factors.[38] However, the complex interplay of genetic and environmental interactions in creating a vulnerability for depression amongst abused children has been demonstrated,[39] and it is likely that similar gene-environment interactions are involved in the development of PTSD.

The politics of PTSD

What are the implications of classifying PTSD as a psychiatric disorder? On the one hand, this classification is important because it acknowledges the severe impact of trauma and indicates that some form of intervention may be required in order to assist the trauma survivor to recover. This gives trauma survivors, often from disempowered groups in society (such as women, children and impoverished communities), access to proper psychiatric and psychological care.[40] On the other hand, some authors have argued that people with PTSD should not be pathologised as having a mental disorder.

40

Young[41] and Summerfield[42] have traced the cultural, historical and political factors that gave impetus to the development of PTSD as a diagnostic category, highlighting the shifting nature of our understandings of 'traumatic stress' and the ways in which, over the past century, it has come to be socially constructed as an 'illness' rather than as a normal and appropriate response to abnormal experiences. Summerfield argues that since the majority of trauma victims tend to be politically oppressed and/or economically impoverished, trauma and its effects are symptoms of power imbalances in society, not of individual disorder.[43] He strongly disputes the inclusion of such social suffering within the domain of biological psychiatry, arguing that 'distress or suffering is not psychopathology'.[44] This medicalisation of suffering, while offering a form of acknowledgement to victims, has potentially conservative ideological implications, for it offers an apolitical and de-contextualised understanding of trauma. This may serve to de-legitimise experiences of oppression and exploitation, to marginalise survivors' feelings of outrage and injustice and to relegate responsibility for trauma recovery to the individual and those offering individually oriented interventions, rather than to broader societal structures.[45] In this way, constructing PTSD as an individual mental disorder ultimately leads to the maintenance of social inequalities.

From a bio-medical perspective, the argument that PTSD is not a form of individual psychopathology is not well supported by the available evidence. The research findings that PTSD affects only a minority of trauma survivors and that the neurobiological functioning of survivors with PTSD is qualitatively different from those without PTSD suggest that PTSD constitutes a disruption of, or deviation from, the normal stress response. This does not imply that the trauma survivor is somehow to blame for their symptoms, but it does imply that some form of individual intervention may be required to help the survivor to regain their best possible functioning in the world.

The current polarisation between the psychiatric and social perspectives on PTSD is important for stimulating debate and further research on trauma responses, but often tends to reduce an extremely complex issue to an either/or dichotomy. The phenomenon of PTSD clearly has both bio-medical and social aspects, and an integrated understanding of both is necessary in order to do justice to the needs of trauma survivors.[46] The cultural dominance of any one particular discourse or perspective on PTSD needs to be carefully interrogated by researchers and clinicians, who ultimately produce the published knowledge base about trauma.

Other Disorders Associated with PTSD

Responses to trauma are highly complex, and posttraumatic symptoms may not be restricted to those characterised by PTSD. Research in the United States indicates that the majority (some studies suggest as much as 80–90 per cent) of trauma survivors who develop PTSD also have other psychiatric disorders.[47] The psychiatric disorders that are commonly comorbid with PTSD (in other words, that occur together with PTSD), and that are commonly found amongst trauma survivors who do not develop PTSD, include mood disorders, phobias and substance abuse.

Mood disorders that often occur together with PTSD include depression and dysthymia. Almost half of the trauma survivors who have PTSD also have depression.[48] In addition, many survivors who do not develop PTSD after a traumatic experience do go on to develop depression.[49] The clinical picture of depression consists of low mood and/or loss of interest or pleasure in regular activities, together with appetite and sleep disturbances, restlessness or agitation, fatigue or low energy, feelings of worthlessness or guilt, loss of concentration, and possibly suicidal thoughts. These symptoms must be present most of the day, nearly every day, for at least two weeks, and must result in significant distress or noticeable impairment in the person's daily functioning.[50] Dysthymia refers to a milder but more chronic form of depression that lasts for at least two years.[51]

Phobias that commonly occur after trauma include a phobia of specific objects or places (which may be associated with the trauma experience), social phobia (a fear and avoidance of social situations because of anxiety about being evaluated and judged negatively by others) and agoraphobia (fear of being in spaces from which one could not easily escape in the event of having panic-like symptoms, which often leads to an avoidance of leaving home alone for any reason).

In North American studies, between 65–80 per cent of patients seeking treatment for PTSD also have a substance abuse disorder.[52] Substance abuse disorders may include the abuse of alcohol, prescription medication or other drugs, to a degree that results in significant distress or impairment in functioning (for example, difficulty fulfilling work or home obligations, or engaging in dangerous behaviours while intoxicated).[53] It is possible that people with PTSD or other posttraumatic symptoms may use substances to try to manage their distress and anxiety, a pattern known as self-medication.

There are still some unanswered questions regarding the exact nature of the relationship between PTSD and other disorders that are commonly found amongst trauma survivors. For example, we do not yet know for certain whether pre-existing mood, anxiety and substance abuse disorders create a vulnerability that increases the likelihood of developing PTSD after a trauma, whether the distressing experience of having PTSD itself results in depressed mood, phobias and substance abuse, or whether PTSD and its comorbid disorders develop separately from each other after a trauma. However, the available information suggests that mood disorders and substance abuse tend to develop after PTSD, while phobias and other anxiety disorders sometimes (but not always) pre-date PTSD and may create a vulnerability for PTSD after trauma exposure.[54] Another issue is that there is a large amount of overlap between the symptoms of PTSD and the symptoms of depression, dysthymia and phobias. For example, social withdrawal is one of the avoidance symptoms of PTSD, but also a primary symptom of depression, dysthymia, social phobia and agoraphobia. Similarly, concentration and sleep difficulties are symptoms of PTSD but also of depression and dysthymia. It is therefore difficult to establish whether depression, phobias and substance abuse are distinct and separate disorders from PTSD, or are all part of a broad posttraumatic syndrome. Nevertheless, it is apparent that posttraumatic symptoms often extend beyond those captured by the PTSD diagnosis, creating multiple difficulties and challenges for many trauma survivors.

The Effects of Prolonged Trauma Exposure or Abuse

Since PTSD first entered the psychiatric classification system in 1980, it has become increasingly apparent to researchers and clinicians that the psychological effects of being in a situation of chronic, repeated trauma at the hands of another person over a long period of time (such as childhood physical or sexual abuse, abuse by an intimate partner, or war captivity) are different to the effects of a single trauma such as a violent crime or serious car accident. Researchers in economically developed countries such as the United States of America and the United Kingdom have reported that many survivors of chronic trauma or abuse perpetrated by a loved and trusted person (such as a parent figure or an intimate partner) present with patterns of difficulties that do not fit with the classic PTSD symptoms.[55] The syndromes of 'complex PTSD',[56] 'disorders of extreme stress not otherwise specified' (DESNOS)[57] and 'enduring personality changes after catastrophic experience'[58] have been proposed and elaborated by North American, British and European researchers to describe the impact of prolonged traumatisation. These syndromes describe the way that survivors of chronic trauma feel about themselves, their characteristic patterns of managing difficult feelings and their relationship styles.

Survivors of early or chronic abuse often experience a disturbed sense of personal identity, ranging from feelings of fragmentation (for example, experiencing their feelings as being foreign, uncontrollable and frightening), feeling completely detached from themselves, or even feeling that they do not really exist. In addition, the survivor might have experiences of alterations in consciousness, including periods of dissociation – that is, 'blanking out' and not being aware afterwards of what he or she said or did while in this state. Dissociative Identity Disorder,[59] which used to be known as Multiple Personality Disorder, is a rare and extreme form of dissociation in which distinct personalities develop in the person's psyche, and it is usually a consequence of chronic and severe early child abuse. Experiences of detachment and dissociation initially develop as protective internal coping mechanisms to enable the person to psychologically 'remove' themselves from chronically traumatic experiences that they cannot physically escape, but these mechanisms create ongoing difficulties in the long term.

Survivors of prolonged trauma, especially at the hands of a controlling abuser, may also carry feelings of helplessness and passivity, of not being able to take initiative in acting on the environment. In addition, survivors of abuse (especially abuse perpetrated in close relationships) often blame themselves rather than the perpetrator for what took place. It is much easier to believe that they are bad and deserving of abuse than to believe that a loved one has chosen to hurt them.[60] This may result in powerful feelings of guilt, shame and unworthiness, and the survivor may view himself or herself as unlovable, despicable and weak, and possibly as evil or contaminated.

Survivors of chronic trauma also display a marked difficulty with regulating or controlling strong feelings, such as sadness or anger, resulting in unpredictable emotional outbursts. They often have an inability to soothe themselves, and may even struggle to derive comfort from supportive others. This results in potentially harmful strategies for managing feelings of distress or anger, such as substance abuse, eating disorders, secretly cutting oneself in order to release emotional tension, and attempting suicide. For survivors of abuse, emotional distress may often manifest itself bodily in somatic symptoms – that is, in physical complaints that have no medical basis. For example, many survivors of childhood sexual abuse experience chronic pelvic pain, gastrointestinal discomfort and numbing or paralysis in different parts of their body with no medical explanation.[61] These symptoms are understood to be the result of a conversion of emotional distress into bodily pain.

The relationship patterns that develop as a result of prolonged traumatisation at the hands of another person tend to further exacerbate the trauma survivor's difficulties in living. Survivors of abuse may have extreme difficulty with trusting others, resulting in social isolation and withdrawal. Alternatively, out of a need for love and acceptance, the survivor may trust other people indiscriminately, or become excessively accommodating of other people's needs in order to prevent abandonment by them. Together with their chronic feelings of unworthiness, self-blame and inherent badness, this can result in the survivor being repeatedly emotionally or physically abused by others.

Indeed, research has found that women who were sexually abused in childhood are more than twice as likely to be sexually abused in adulthood than women who experienced no childhood sexual abuse.[62]

Why do many survivors of early childhood abuse develop what has been called 'complex PTSD' (although given the substantial differences from classic PTSD, these symptoms could perhaps more accurately be called 'complex traumatic stress reactions')? Neurobiological and developmental research has begun to map the ways in which early childhood trauma shapes the development of the emerging brain.[63] Repeated traumatic experiences in childhood 'train' the brain to focus on responding to danger and threat rather than to focus on learning and exploration. Those neural pathways that govern defensive responses to danger or threat therefore become overdeveloped, while those that are responsible for other tasks (including the capacity for trust, the expression of emotions through language, and flexible adaptation to change or stress in the environment) remain underdeveloped. In particular, traumatised children often do not develop the neural networks that assist with the capacity for secure attachment and for identifying and thinking about their needs and feelings without simply acting on them. As a result, patterns of response to the early traumatic situation become entrenched and continue into adulthood, even when the abusive situation may longer be ongoing. Without the capacity for secure and trusting attachments, or for reflective self-awareness, survivors of childhood abuse are often at risk of re-creating abusive relationships in adulthood.

Because the psychological effects of early or prolonged abuse are extremely complex, and can differ substantially from more classic PTSD symptoms, clinicians and counsellors often find it difficult to accurately diagnose those survivors of abuse who present themselves for help. This is exacerbated by the fact that many such survivors, due to deep feelings of shame or distrust, do not actually disclose their experiences of abuse to those who are treating them. As a result, such patients are often diagnosed with a mixed bag of different disorders, in order to account for their many and varied symptoms, or with a personality disorder such as Borderline Personality Disorder.[64] Such patients often return again and again for help, but may repeatedly fail to be correctly identified as trauma survivors by the mental health system. That is why the recent concepts of 'complex PTSD' and 'disorders of extreme stress not otherwise specified' are extremely useful clinical tools for understanding the needs of survivors of abuse. See Box 3.3 below for an illustrative case study of complex PTSD.

Box 3.3 Case study of complex PTSD

Joy is a 24-year-old woman living with a female flatmate in Johannesburg. She was admitted to a psychiatric hospital after a suicide attempt. During the interview with the clinician it emerged that, as a child, Joy was sexually abused by her stepfather from the age of 7 years old (when he first moved into the house with her and her mother) until the age of 15 years, when Joy went to live with her biological father in another city. At the time, Joy told no one about the abuse, including her mother who she felt was very emotionally fragile and would not be able to cope with the situation. Since childhood, Joy has struggled with feelings of worthlessness and not being good enough. Although she has attempted to study several different courses at university and has had a number of different casual jobs to earn money, she always feels that she is not doing well enough and is incapable of being a success at anything, and gives up after a few months. Her social life is also very unstable, as she tends to make friends very quickly with people but then soon finds herself feeling let down and rejected by them, becomes angry with them, and withdraws herself from the relationship. In order to cope with her feelings of emptiness, rejection and worthlessness, she drinks several glasses of wine every evening and also smokes marijuana several times a week. She has had several brief romantic relationships with men who are much older than herself, but in each case she has felt 'treated like an object' by them – she feels that they use her for their own needs but are not really interested in her needs. However, she is never the one to end these relationships – rather 'they just dump me when they'd had enough'. On several occasions when she has felt very distressed, such as when she was fired from a casual job due to repeated absences, or when a man she had been dating broke up with her without explanation, she has cut herself on her legs with a piece of broken glass from a mirror 'just to give myself some relief from my feelings'. Recently she has been having a relationship with a married man. During an argument with him last week, Joy says she became so angry she 'blanked out', and when she became aware of herself again she found herself physically attacking him. He then told Joy she was 'crazy' and he didn't want to see her ever again. That night Joy took an overdose of sleeping tablets. Her flatmate found her shortly thereafter and called an ambulance.

The Effects of Community Violence: A Continuous Traumatic Stress Syndrome?

The development of the concepts of 'complex PTSD' or 'disorders of extreme stress' represents a significant advance in our knowledge about the effects of trauma, and addresses some of the diagnostic confusion that has existed with regard to survivors of early or prolonged trauma and abuse. These concepts capture the complex psychological impact of being abused repeatedly, in a predictable but uncontrollable way, by the same perpetrator over a period of time, and provide some understanding of why many survivors of childhood abuse find themselves in similarly abusive relationship patterns in adulthood.

However, these concepts also have some limitations. Situations of prolonged abuse at the hands of another person need to be distinguished from another type of prolonged traumatisation which is characteristic of many economically disadvantaged communities in South Africa and other countries. This involves repeated exposure to community violence on a daily basis, including gang violence and gun warfare in one's neighbourhood, school violence, and opportunistic criminal assaults and sexual assaults. As we have seen in the previous chapter, for many South Africans this continuous community violence is exacerbated by physical, emotional or sexual abuse occurring in the home, with the victims being primarily women and children.

A vast number of South Africans therefore do not enjoy a sense of physical safety and security either at home or outside the home, and often have been victimised by multiple perpetrators of violence, some of whom may be familiar (such as a spouse or neighbour) and some of whom may be total strangers. The occurrence of violence is therefore common yet unpredictable with regard to where it may happen, what form it might take and who the perpetrator might be. A person living in a highly violent community must not only deal with their own experiences of direct traumatisation, but also with the indirect trauma of hearing gunshots and seeing weapons in the neighbourhood, witnessing others being assaulted, and hearing about the violence experienced by family members, neighbours and friends. This is further exacerbated by the constant anxiety of worrying about the safety of themselves and their loved ones. Finally, for many South Africans, the stress of living in conditions of continuous traumatisation is compounded by the chronic uncertainty and anxiety wrought by severe economic deprivation.

It could therefore be argued that many South Africans do not have a 'post'-trauma period in which to process, or attempt to adapt to, their recent trauma experiences, before the next traumatic experience (whether it is direct or indirect) occurs. The psychological effects of this form of cumulative and continuous trauma, as distinct from repeated abuse at the hands of someone known to the victim, are not well documented in the international literature. In the 1980s, a group of South African therapists working with anti-apartheid activists suffering ongoing state repression, often in hiding or on the run, and facing detention without trial, interrogation or worse, coined the term 'continuous traumatic stress' to represent the fact that for these clients danger was not past (or 'post') and that they faced ongoing risk of further traumatisation.[65] Although this context of political activism and state repression has passed, this term still has enormous relevance to the many communities in South Africa where trauma exposure is an inescapable part of daily life. However, the characteristics of continuous traumatic stress have never really been fully investigated and described and, as we shall see in the next section, South African research has yet to tackle the question of how the psychological impact of continuous community trauma differs from the impact of single traumas or of an ongoing abusive relationship.

South African Research On The Psychiatric Effects Of Trauma

A wealth of knowledge about the impact of trauma has emerged in South Africa over the past few decades. At the same time, there are some aspects that remain poorly understood and require further attention. Studies conducted with South African adults will be considered here, while studies of the impact of trauma on South African children and adolescents will be discussed in Chapter 6.

South African research on the effects of trauma emerged during the 1980s within the context of political violence under apartheid. However, given the scope and scale of political violence in South Africa during this time (see Chapter 2), and the range of interventions that were being offered to survivors of political violence by those counsellors committed to social activism, surprisingly little research on the psychological impact of state-sponsored violence was published. This was likely due not only to the conservative ideological and political stance of mainstream organised psychology in South Africa during the apartheid years,[66] but also to the very challenging conditions under which those trauma counsellors who were treating survivors of political violence had to work. For example, raids of counselling centres by police or political vigilantes were common in the 1980s.[67] Working in a perpetual crisis mode left little space for politically progressive psychologists to conduct and write up systematic research on the effects of political violence, although some of the experiences of working with detainees and other victims of state repression were documented in the South Africa-based journal *Psychology in Society*. Published research on the effects of state-sponsored violence during the 1980s and early 1990s focused mainly on children and youth (see Chapter 6), while very little research on work with adult survivors was published. As noted in Chapter 1, much of the rich knowledge base that developed during this time was shared and documented in other, less formal ways.

Perhaps the largest and most systematic study of the psychological impact of organised state violence on South African adults was completed by Foster and his colleagues in 1987.[68] They conducted semi-structured interviews with 176 political prisoners in detention, of whom 83 per cent reported that they had been physically tortured. While the diagnosis of PTSD was not assessed in this sample, these prisoners commonly reported symptoms of anxiety, depression, impaired cognitive functioning, somatisation and emotional numbing. Another study of ninety-five participants who had been displaced as the result of political violence in KwaZulu Natal in 1990 found that 87 per cent reported symptoms of PTSD, and that such symptoms were highest amongst those who witnessed a friend or family member being killed.[69]

More recently, several studies have assessed the long-term impact of political violence by assessing the psychological well-being of survivors in the post-apartheid era. In general, these studies have reported high rates of psychiatric disorders. For example, in 1998 a DSM-IV-based psychiatric interview (a structured interview assessing a variety of psychiatric disorders using the diagnostic criteria that are specified in the American Psychiatric Association's *Diagnostic and Statistical Manual of Mental Disorders, Fourth Edition* [DSM-IV; APA, 2000]) was used to assess fourteen South African torture survivors presenting at an anxiety disorders clinic. The study found that all of the participants had PTSD and panic disorder, while 57 per cent met the diagnostic criteria for depression.[70] Another study with 147 survivors of human rights abuses presenting for psychological services in KwaZulu-Natal utilised a semi-structured screening questionnaire for psychological disorders, as well as a PTSD symptom checklist.[71] Rates of PTSD varied across geographical areas but were generally high (ranging from 25–56 per cent), while anxiety disorders, depression, substance abuse and somatic complaints were also common. A Cape Town study recruited 134 volunteer participants from community settings who had experienced human rights abuses.[72] Using a structured psychiatric interview, the study found that 55 per cent of the participants had depression, 42 per cent had PTSD, 27 per cent had another anxiety disorder, and 54 per cent had more than one psychiatric diagnosis. Furthermore, somatic complaints such as bodily pains with no medical basis were also common in this sample.[73] Another study with twenty ex-detainees used a semi-structured qualitative interview to elicit participants' own reports about their current concerns.[74] The study found that the most pressing concerns for these survivors of political violence were, in order of importance, somatic complaints, economic stressors, dissatisfaction with the political dispensation in South Africa, and symptoms of posttraumatic stress that were not always severe enough to warrant a diagnosis of PTSD. Research with ex-combatants from a number of different military structures found that the majority of interviewees reported experiencing a range of PTSD symptoms, such as flashbacks and nightmares. In addition, many of them reported related difficulties such as substance abuse and aggressive outbursts.[75]

On the whole, these clinic and community-based studies indicate that survivors of political violence in South Africa continue to have many unmet mental health needs. However, it could be argued that the strength of these findings is limited by some methodological issues. It is not possible from these studies to conclusively show that experiences of political violence have been the direct cause of psychiatric disorders like PTSD and depression, since many other factors (such as other traumas or life stressors) may have played a causal role. In addition, these studies utilised samples that may not be very representative of all survivors of political violence. For example, some of the participants in these studies were patients attending clinics for treatment. Others had volunteered to participate in the study in response to advertisements or word-of-mouth requests, but may have had specific motivations for volunteering. The SASH survey allowed for a somewhat more systematic investigation of the link between political violence and psychiatric disorder. In this large nationally representative sample, it was found that, among men, experiences of detention and torture carried the highest risk for PTSD compared with a range of other forms of violence.[76] This finding confirms that political violence does indeed have a strong link with PTSD, although it does not exclude the possibility that other factors may also play a role.

We have seen in Chapter 2 that many South Africans have been and continue to be exposed to criminal violence, either directly or indirectly. Despite this, there is surprisingly little South African research on the effects of criminal violence on mental health. One study with a sample of adult victims of violent crime (including sexual assaults, armed robberies and attempted murders) in Pietersburg used two different PTSD symptom self-report scales to assess the rate of PTSD symptoms.[77] The percentage of participants who were at high risk for having PTSD was 25 per cent on the one scale and 42 per cent on the other scale. Another study using interviews to qualitatively explore the effects of hijackings on four victims also reported some PTSD symptoms.[78] These two studies suggest that many victims of violent crime might experience symptoms of posttraumatic stress but, since neither study used standardised psychiatric interviews, they could not establish how many participants actually met the full diagnostic criteria for PTSD. In the SASH survey,[79] which used a psychiatric interview to establish whether the full diagnosis of PTSD was met, criminal violence had a low association with PTSD amongst men, compared with many other kinds of violence (such as torture or childhood physical abuse).

But for women, non-sexual criminal violence was more than twice as likely to be associated with PTSD as it was for men.

The psychiatric impact of gender-based violence has very seldom been systematically researched in South Africa, despite the scale and severity of gender-based violence in this country. In one study of 1,050 female patients visiting general practitioners, assessment with self-report questionnaires found that 35 per cent of those who had experienced domestic violence were at high risk of having a diagnosis of PTSD, compared with only 3 per cent of those who had not experienced domestic violence.[80] Rates of depressive symptoms were also substantially higher among those women who were survivors of domestic violence. Another study with 250 rape survivors reported moderate levels of re-experiencing, avoidance and hyperarousal symptoms, with hyperarousal predominating slightly. The participants also reported behavioural changes such as social withdrawal and avoidant styles of coping.[81] Consistent with findings in other countries, the SASH national survey found that rape carries the highest risk for PTSD amongst women, followed by intimate partner violence.[82] Given the prevalence and the high degree of toxicity of gender-based violence, more research is urgently needed in order to fully understand the mental health needs of the many women and girls in South Africa who have experienced sexual and physical violence.

With the high prevalence of HIV/AIDS in South Africa,[83] it is important to understand the mental health impact of receiving this diagnosis. While psychiatric disorders are only one aspect of the multiple psychological challenges presented by living with HIV/AIDS, they cannot be neglected since psychiatric disorders like depression may affect the course of HIV infection[84] and may also reduce the HIV-positive person's adherence to a treatment regimen.[85] One study followed up a group of fifty-one HIV-positive women in Cape Town over a six-month period, and found that depression and PTSD were the most common psychiatric disorders, both at the first interview (34.9 per cent for depression and 14.8 per cent for PTSD) and six months later at the second (26 per cent for depression and 20 per cent for PTSD).[86] While there was a substantial increase in the number of participants meeting criteria for PTSD over this period, this study could not directly establish a link between receiving an HIV-positive diagnosis and the development of subsequent PTSD. A study with 465 participants receiving treatment for HIV/AIDS in Cape Town reported that 14 per cent of the sample met criteria for depression, 5 per cent met criteria for PTSD and 7 per cent met criteria for substance abuse.[87] Again, the study could not establish whether there was a causal relationship between receiving a diagnosis of HIV/AIDS and the development of these psychiatric disorders. However, another study of recently diagnosed HIV-positive patients in the Western Cape found that 40 per cent of the sample had PTSD specifically linked to receiving an HIV diagnosis or to being HIV-positive.[88] This suggests a more direct casual relationship between hearing about one's HIV-positive status and the development of PTSD.

Although rates of traffic injuries are high in South Africa, as discussed in the previous chapter, there is a lack of research documenting the psychiatric impact of such accidental trauma. Using self-report instruments, one study reported that people involved in traffic accidents as drivers or as passengers experience a significant decrease in their general health and quality of life after the accident, and also experience a high rate of post-traumatic symptoms like avoidance and intrusive recollections.[89] But other studies of psychiatric symptoms among South Africans who have been involved in traffic injuries are scarce. Given that claims for compensation for road accident injuries are often made on the basis of a resulting psychiatric disorder, some prevalence data on the psychiatric impact of traffic accidents in our population would be valuable.

Some research has been conducted with samples that are routinely exposed to trauma as part of their occupations. For example, using a psychiatric interview and self-report questionnaires with 198 members of the South African National Defence Force, one study found that 25 per cent currently met the criteria for PTSD and 17 per cent were at high risk for receiving a diagnosis of depression.[90] Several studies with members of the South African Police have similarly found a high rate of symptoms typical of PTSD,[91] although the use of self-report scales rather than psychiatric interviews limited the degree to which rates of full-blown PTSD could be ascertained. Research on the mental health needs of people working in occupations with a high risk of exposure to life-threatening events is important in order to motivate for them to have better access to mental health resources.

A few studies have examined posttraumatic symptoms among patients presenting at primary health care clinics in South Africa. One study used a psychiatric interview to assess 201 patients at an urban township clinic in Cape Town, and found that 19.9 per cent had a current diagnosis of PTSD, but that depression and somatisation disorder were also very common and were frequently comorbid with PTSD.[92] Using a self-report questionnaire, a study with clinic patients in a rural area of South Africa found that 12.4 per cent were at high risk of having PTSD, but other diagnoses were not assessed.[93]

To date, the SASH survey is the only South African study to examine the prevalence of PTSD in the South African population as a whole, using a DSM-IV-based standardised psychiatric interview (the Composite International Diagnostic Interview Version 3.0 or CIDI).[94] Interestingly, this survey found a very low rate of PTSD nationally compared with that reported in many other countries. In the SASH sample, the lifetime prevalence rate of PTSD (that is, the percentage of the sample that had ever had a diagnosis of PTSD in their lifetime) was 2.3 per cent,[95] compared with around 8–9 per cent in the American population[96] and 11.2 per cent in the Mexican population,[97] both of which have rates of trauma exposure that are similar to those found in South Africa. However, it would be premature to conclude from this that South Africans are not severely affected by trauma. Firstly, the SASH finding of a low rate of PTSD in the South African population may be the result of issues in the translation of the standardised diagnostic interview into six different South African languages, possibly affecting the way in which questions about symptoms were understood by respondents. Secondly, the effects of trauma in the South African population may be different to those that have been documented in countries such as the United States, where the DSM-IV was developed. The SASH study also assessed levels of general distress in the sample (for example, feeling nervous, irritable, depressed and fatigued), as opposed to specific psychiatric disorders, and found that levels of distress increased dramatically with more exposure to trauma: those

South Africans who had experienced six or more traumas were five times more likely to have high distress than individuals who had experienced no traumas.[98] This suggests a cumulative negative emotional effect of trauma exposure among South Africans, lending support to the notion of a continuous traumatic stress response that may not necessarily be manifested as PTSD.

In sum, studies with South African trauma survivors have tended to focus on establishing the presence of symptoms of PTSD and, sometimes, depression, in keeping with international research which has demonstrated that these disorders are commonly found amongst trauma survivors. Local studies have consistently found very high levels of PTSD and depressive symptomatology across various groups of trauma survivors, suggesting that these are very common responses to trauma exposure in our population, and that substantial mental health resources need to be allocated to address these issues. However, we must still remain somewhat cautious about drawing this conclusion. In many cases, studies have relied on self-report questionnaires which do not indicate whether symptoms are of sufficient duration and severity to warrant a clinical diagnosis, and can, in fact, overestimate the prevalence of disorder.[99] More time-consuming and costly research using structured psychiatric interviews is needed in order to better understand the mental health needs of trauma survivors. The nationally representative SASH survey, which used a psychiatric interview to assess the presence of PTSD, indicated that rates of full-blown PTSD (that is, PTSD symptoms that are enduring, cause substantial distress, and significantly reduce the person's ability to function) may, in fact, be quite low amongst trauma survivors in South Africa. However, not all structured psychiatric interviews are necessarily useful in the local context. There is some interesting preliminary evidence from a six-month follow-up study of rape survivors in Cape Town that, even when participants are assessed in their first language, their response to questions about PTSD symptoms varies substantially depending on how exactly the questions are phrased.[100] Given our many indigenous languages, we still have some way to go in establishing exactly which instruments are most valid and reliable for assessing posttraumatic symptoms in our population.

Another limitation of the existing research is that it tends to be cross-sectional (assessing a sample at one specific point in time), which makes it difficult to conclusively establish a causal link between a past trauma and current symptoms. Although the SASH study established that certain types of trauma (specifically, torture for men and rape for women) have a stronger association with PTSD, the prevalence of multiple trauma exposure in our population makes it difficult to causally link one particular kind of past trauma with current PTSD symptoms. It is also possible that current symptoms of depression frequently reported by South African trauma survivors may in fact pre-date exposure to a trauma. Longitudinal research that follows up a group of participants over a period of time would help to clarify the causal relationships between different types of trauma exposure and different psychiatric symptoms.

Since increased trauma exposure amongst South Africans is strongly related to an increase in levels of general distress, it is likely that many trauma survivors in South Africa experience psychiatric symptoms that are, in fact, sub-clinical, or below the threshold for diagnosis. These sub-clinical symptoms may nonetheless reduce the quality of life of trauma survivors in numerous ways. It also seems possible that responses to trauma in the South African population may fit more closely with other types of diagnoses, besides PTSD and depression. For example, it is interesting to note that when South African researchers have attempted to explore the psychiatric effects of trauma more broadly, somatic symptoms appear to be commonly reported. This is consistent with findings from a study with traumatised Sudanese refugees in Uganda and torture survivors in Malawi,[101] and suggests that the impact of trauma amongst South Africans and those living in other countries in Africa may be more extensive than what emerges from a narrow focus on PTSD or depression.

There are still many aspects of the effects of trauma in South Africa that need to be better understood. For example, despite South Africa's high rates of child sexual and physical abuse and intimate partner abuse, we still know very little about the psychiatric effects of prolonged abuse in our population. Although the SASH survey established that exposure to multiple traumas is associated with more severe levels of general distress, the specific psychiatric consequences of multiple traumatisation and continuous community violence still remain unclear. Finally, South African studies have seldom explored whether the psychiatric consequences of trauma are associated with socio-economic status. The particular ways in which conditions of poverty may impact upon coping after trauma need further exploration, if we are to provide effective support to trauma survivors who may be disempowered at a number of levels.

Conclusion

Many trauma survivors are able to return to their normal functioning within a few days or weeks after a traumatic event. However, as a result of the interaction of a number of factors, some survivors develop a more long-lasting set of symptoms that may fit the diagnostic picture of PTSD. While PTSD has received a lot of attention in the media and popular culture, depression, phobias and substance abuse are also common psychiatric consequences of trauma. In the South African context, most research with trauma survivors has focused quite narrowly on assessing symptoms of PTSD and, to a lesser extent, depression. However, some emerging evidence suggests that other types of symptoms may be quite prevalent amongst South African trauma survivors, particularly somatic symptoms.

In international research, it is increasingly apparent that survivors of early and prolonged abuse often develop difficulties that are not consistent with PTSD or other diagnoses commonly associated with single traumatic events. But the effects of prolonged abuse in South Africa have not yet been well documented and require further exploration. In addition, the psychological impact of living in a highly violent community is not yet well understood. This is an important avenue for research in South Africa, where many people live in contexts of continuous community violence, and there is an opportunity for South African researchers to make a valuable contribution to the international literature in this area.

Psychiatric diagnoses are a useful tool because they alert us to the common and universal aspects of experiences of distress. For example, the diagnosis of PTSD or the more recent syndrome of complex PTSD both highlight symptoms that are shared by many trauma survivors, and thereby serve to normalise and validate their feelings and experiences. But regardless of whether a survivor's response objectively 'fits' a particular posttraumatic diagnosis, the subjective process of trying to adapt to a traumatic experience is unique for each trauma survivor. For example, no two rape survivors with PTSD have exactly the same internal experience of trying to adapt to what has happened to them. The danger of psychiatric diagnoses is that they tend to disguise or silence variations in the subjective experience of distress. In the next chapter, we move beyond a focus on post-trauma psychiatric disorders to explore the ways in which trauma can impact upon our personal systems of meaning, elaborating some of the more clearly psychological theory about the impact of trauma exposure.

Chapter 4

TRAUMA AS A CRISIS
OF MEANING

While much of the psychological literature on the effects of trauma has focused on specific psychiatric symptoms such as PTSD, there has also been increasing recognition that trauma presents an enormous challenge to our belief and meaning systems, even in the absence of PTSD or other symptoms. Survivors of trauma often struggle to develop an understanding of why the trauma happened, and of why they were singled out to be a victim. They may wrestle with how to reconcile the trauma experience with their fundamental expectations and beliefs about themselves, other people, and the world, leaving them feeling vulnerable, distrustful and uncertain. Faced with this existential crisis, trauma survivors try to develop explanations for the traumatic event and to generate meanings that will allow them to make sense of the world in future. Sometimes the explanations and meanings that are generated enable the survivor to re-establish a sense of trust, control and purpose, while in other cases the explanations and meanings that are formed serve to maintain or even exacerbate the survivor's feelings of distrust, lack of control and despair. This chapter will explore what we currently understand about the 'meaning' dimension of the psychological impact of trauma.

Shattered Assumptions and the Search for Comprehensibility

In the previous chapter, we saw that PTSD symptoms of re-experiencing the trauma may occur because traumatic events cannot be categorised and integrated within the beliefs (or schemas) about ourselves, others and the world that we held before the trauma – they simply cannot be located within our existing cognitive map of the world.[1] Janoff-Bulman has identified several core beliefs or assumptions that people hold regarding themselves, others and the world, that are shattered by a traumatic experience.[2] She argues that we all carry implicit assumptions that we take for granted and which we are not always consciously aware of – they are an invisible but vital part of our internal cognitive model of the world and underpin a sense of basic well-being. These include the assumption that we are invulnerable (for example, believing that 'it can't happen to me'), that we are good and worthy people, that other people are fundamentally good, and that the world is governed by just and orderly social laws (for example, 'if I am cautious, I can avoid misfortune', or 'if I am good, nothing bad will happen to me').

Even if we are intellectually aware that our safety and security are not guaranteed, that other people often have hostile intentions and that sometimes bad things happen to good people out of sheer random chance, we still hold the above assumptions at a less conscious level, for these beliefs help us to maintain some sense of predictability and control in a world that would otherwise feel utterly random and unpredictable. Often we are not even aware that we hold such assumptions, until an experience of trauma suddenly makes us realise that we have taken these beliefs for granted and that we now need to profoundly re-examine them.[3] For example, intense feelings of powerlessness during and after a trauma may shatter the survivor's basic trust in their own capacity to control events and themselves. The shattering of assumptions of personal competence and control, and of one's basic trust in the inherent justness, order and benevolence of the universe, creates enormous distress, vulnerability and uncertainty for many trauma survivors.

Other researchers have argued that not all people implicitly hold positive assumptions about themselves, other people and the world – rather, people who have had a history of early trauma or of severe psychological difficulties are more likely to quite rigidly perceive the world as being dangerous, others as untrustworthy and themselves as incompetent and unworthy.[4] For these people, a new experience of trauma serves to confirm, rather than shatter, their pre-existing negative assumptions. Researchers suggest that it is those people whose pre-trauma assumptions are very rigid or extreme, whether in a positive *or* a negative direction, who most struggle to process a trauma experience in a meaningful way. For those who hold very positive assumptions, an experience of trauma violates their existing understandings of the world, leaving a meaning 'vacuum', while for those who hold very negative assumptions, a trauma experience may reinforce their belief that the world is dangerous and unpredictable and that they themselves are unworthy and incompetent. In both cases, the trauma survivor is left with a heightened sense of vulnerability and lack of control.

In their struggle to deal with feelings of uncertainty and vulnerability in the aftermath of trauma, many survivors wrestle with questions such as 'why does this sort of thing happen in the world?', 'how can people do this sort of thing to other people?' and 'why did this happen to me?'.[5] These are not simply rhetorical questions arising out of a sense of despair and disillusionment. Rather, they are active attempts to make the trauma experience more intelligible, and the search for comprehensibility entails an exploration and evaluation of different causal explanations. However, the search for an explanation is not just an intellectual exercise, but also a deeply emotional process that may take trauma survivors through a range of different feelings at different points in time.[6] Searching for meaning is also not always a conscious strategy; survivors do not explicitly tell themselves that they need to rebuild their fundamental assumptions and find an explanation for the trauma. Rather, the process of trying to make sense of the trauma is part of the natural process of seeking to re-establish equilibrium after a crisis.[7]

Why do so many trauma survivors seek an explanation for the trauma? The establishment of causal linkages between events is a central component of any well-formed story,[8] but causal accounts are particularly important for making sense of extraordinary events.[9] The stories we tell each other about our ordinary, everyday experiences often tend to just be descriptive (telling *what* happened) and to not include explanatory accounts (telling *why* it happened). Everyday experiences, fitting as they do with our existing cultural beliefs and expectations, are simply taken for granted. However, in response to extraordinary experiences, such as life traumas, we may be more likely to try to develop not just descriptive but also explanatory stories, in an attempt to formulate a meaningful and comprehensible account of things that deviate substantially from established cultural norms and expectations. While the process of exploring meaningful explanations for a trauma experience is a highly personal process that may take trauma survivors in many different directions, some common explanatory strategies employed by trauma survivors have been documented (see Box 4.1 for a summary). These strategies are attempts to construct models or theories about the world, themselves and other people that enable survivors to make sense of the trauma experience.

How the world works: 'stuff happens' versus 'a greater plan'
In response to being the victim of a traumatic experience such as a criminal assault, a rape, a car accident, a natural disaster, or the diagnosis of a life-threatening illness, trauma survivors often try to develop a theory about how the world or the universe works that adequately explains their being singled out for victimisation.[10] They try to assess whether there are any cause-and-effect laws governing the universe that can explain why they were 'chosen' as a victim and that can guide them as they go forward into the future. Often, the conclusions reached by trauma survivors regarding how the world works fall into one of two opposing positions or philosophies. The first philosophy is that 'stuff happens'. Here the survivor comes to accept that there are no knowable laws and rules that govern how the universe works, that events occur fairly randomly, and that the survivor happened to be the victim of a particular traumatic event due largely to chance, bad luck, or being in the wrong place at the wrong time. For example, in an exploratory study conducted with a group of ten survivors of violent criminal assault who presented to a police station trauma room in Cape Town, half of the survivors believed that chance and bad luck played a major

Box 4.1

Examples of explanatory strategies commonly used by trauma survivors

A. Beliefs about the world:

(1) The trauma was due to random chance or bad luck.

(2) The trauma was part of God's plan.

(3) The trauma was caused by other people using witchcraft.

(4) The trauma was caused by the ancestors because of something I did or did not do.

B. Beliefs about the perpetrator:

(1) The perpetrator did it because s/he is ill or disturbed.

(2) The perpetrator did it because of their social or economic circumstances.

C. Behavioural self-blame:

(1) I was chosen as the victim because I was not careful or vigilant enough.

(2) I was victimised because I did not fight back hard enough.

D. Characterological self-blame:

(1) I was chosen as the victim because I deserve to be punished.

(2) I was chosen as the victim because I am too trusting.

E. Redefining the event and its impact

(1) It could have been worse.

(2) I was lucky compared to some people.

(3) I am coping better than most people would.

role in their victimisation.[11] For some trauma survivors, this conclusion may be comforting because it suggests that they were not specifically singled out by fate for victimisation and did not do anything to deserve suffering or punishment. It therefore preserves a sense of the world as being a fairly benevolent place, most of the time. However, for other trauma survivors, the conclusion that bad things happen randomly and that one can be victimised by chance may exacerbate their sense of unpredictability and vulnerability, as they may feel they have no control over events in their lives.[12]

The second philosophy about how the world works that can be used to explain a traumatic experience is that the trauma was part of some greater plan which cannot be fully known by the survivor.[13] This approach is often informed by religious, spiritual and/or traditional cultural beliefs that the survivor may have held before the trauma, or which they begin to develop after surviving a trauma. Survivors may explain the trauma by drawing on conceptions of God, ancestors in the spirit world, fate, *karma* or destiny. Within these frameworks, the trauma is often conceived of as a deliberate test or task which has been placed in the survivor's path to challenge their belief system, to teach them something or give them insight, or to punish them for some wrongdoing and put them back on the right path.[14] For example, when asked retrospectively how they understood the event and its impact on their lives, 79 per cent of a sample of survivors of the 1993 St. James Church massacre in Cape Town (in which armed members of a political grouping entered the church during a service, killing several congregants and injuring many more) stated that they believed the event was part of God's plan and that He meant them to learn something from the experience.[15] This is perhaps expectable in a sample of church-going participants, but even trauma survivors who are not particularly religious may draw on a spiritual framework to make sense of their experience. For example, 40 per cent of a small sample of South African mothers who had lost a child to cancer, when asked how they have made sense of why such bereavements happen, described a belief in a 'greater scheme' or 'bigger picture' whereby everybody's time to die is pre-determined.[16] Although this did not mean that they felt a sense of acceptance regarding their loss, it was important for them to be able to understand their suffering as being part of a broader, if mysterious, system that had some logic and coherence to it. On the other hand, the experience of trauma can result in a profound shattering of long-held faith and belief systems, and trauma survivors may begin to question the existence of the God, gods or spiritual forces that they previously believed in, resulting in a 'crisis of faith' that is not resolved.[17]

The Hindu concept of *karma* is based on the belief that events may occur in order to balance out one's past actions and experiences (including those that happened in a previous life or incarnation), and that current experiences will be balanced out in a future life or incarnation. Within this belief framework, a traumatic experience may be viewed in two ways, both explanations based on notions of cause-and-effect: either as being the outcome of previous actions and experiences or as something negative that will be balanced out by something more positive in the future.[18] This belief system provides an explanation for why the person has been 'chosen' to experience something extremely adverse and difficult. Similarly, many people in Africa, including many South Africans, believe in a fluid interaction between the natural world and the supernatural world where deceased ancestors reside and from which they continue to exert influence over the living. Within this belief system, traumatic events can be caused by ancestors in the spirit world. A person may be chosen by the ancestors to suffer adversity because that person is in a state of spiritual pollution (related, for example, to certain reproductive activities and cycles, as well as to being in a state of bereavement) and has failed to observe the necessary taboos and rituals to protect him or herself and others from the effects of this[19] or has failed to perform the abeyances expected by ancestors more generally. Furthermore, this cosmology encompasses a belief that witchcraft can be intentionally employed by people to cause distress and suffering for others; traumatic events may therefore also be the outcome of deliberate magical causation by others in one's community.[20]

While the nature of cultural or religious belief systems about how the world works may differ, they all offer a framework of causes and consequences that people can draw on to make sense of events in their lives, including trauma. However, the extent to which individual trauma survivors choose to draw on available cultural and religious belief systems to make meaning out of their experience depends on the survivor's own personality characteristics and prior life experiences. Furthermore, when survivors are familiar with both traditional African cosmologies and Westernised belief systems, as is often the case in South Africa, they may draw on a blend of belief systems while grappling with the meaning of a traumatic experience.[21] Clearly not all trauma survivors from the same religious or ethnic group will develop the same kind of meanings out of their trauma experiences – again, post-trauma meaning-making is a deeply personal process.

Making sense of why other people are violent

When trauma involves some kind of interpersonal violence, rather than an accident or natural disaster, a central struggle for the survivor is the need to understand why another person would intentionally inflict harm on him or her.[22] Consequently, the survivor's search for causal explanations may often focus on the intentional state of the perpetrator, in order to find a comprehensible reason for the perpetrator's actions.

For example, a Canadian study with survivors of incest found that many participants attempted to make sense of their experience by understanding the parental dynamics that had caused the abuse to occur (for example, marital difficulties or their fathers' characterological defects), and that those who had developed such explanatory accounts demonstrated less psychological distress and better social adjustment than those who did not.[23] Similarly, a study with ten female rape survivors attending a rape counselling centre in Cape Town found that most of the participants had managed to develop an explanatory account for the rapist's actions.[24] For example, they viewed the rapist as disturbed or ill, as having a problem with sex, as having a hatred of women, or as having a need for power and control. However, these participants had received some post-rape counselling, which had provided them with a space to explore and develop these explanatory accounts, an opportunity that many trauma survivors do not have.

The need to understand the motivations of the perpetrator is also a concern for survivors of human rights abuses. A study of survivors of human rights violations in South Africa found 'a strong yearning for contact with the people who had caused their suffering' in order to better understand the behaviour of the perpetrators.[25] Similarly, many people who testified before the South African TRC stated a desire to meet with the perpetrators who had harmed them or killed their family members, in order to understand why they had acted as they did.[26]

The study of crime survivors in Cape Town cited earlier in this chapter found that most of these survivors had managed to generate explanations for why people rob and steal from others (for example, due to poverty, oppression, to support a drug habit, as part of gang culture and so on) but that they struggled to develop an explanation for the perpetrator's use of violence and aggression during the criminal assault.[27] They viewed the perpetrator's use of violence as gratuitous and unnecessary in the context of the assault because there was no real threat to the perpetrator – in every case the crime victim had complied with the perpetrator's instructions. Failure to understand the perpetrator's use of violence was a source of ongoing emotional distress for these survivors and led them to question whether they should stay in South Africa, a dilemma that was particularly painful for those participants who had played an active role in the struggle to end apartheid.

Self-Blame

Explanations for why a trauma happened often need to address not only the reasons that the perpetrator did what they did, but also why the survivor was 'selected' to be a victim. The need to understand 'why me?' is important even for survivors of traumas that do not involve interpersonal violence, such as survivors of natural disasters and accidents and those who have a life-threatening illness such as cancer or HIV/AIDS. In trying to make sense of why a traumatic event happened to them, survivors may come to believe that it occurred because of something they did or something that they failed to do. Because assumptions about being competent and in control of things may be deeply challenged by the experience of trauma, survivors often feel ashamed by their failure to prevent the trauma from happening, or even that they are somehow to blame for the trauma.[28] This tendency towards self-blame in order to make sense of why the trauma happened is sometimes exacerbated by blaming reactions from other people, who may find it more comfortable to blame the victim (for example, by telling a crime survivor 'you shouldn't have been walking alone at night' or telling someone with HIV 'you should have been more careful') than to have their own illusions of safety and security challenged.[29]

Janoff-Bulman has identified two forms of self-blame that trauma survivors may use when trying to develop an explanation for why the trauma happened.[30] Behavioural self-blame refers to the survivor's tendency to attribute the trauma to certain behaviours that he or she engaged in or failed to engage in. For example, rape survivors often retrospectively blame themselves for behaviours such as going back to the rapist's apartment or getting into his car, question whether they unwittingly gave the rapist some signal of sexual attraction or wonder whether the rape could have been avoided if they had fought back hard enough. These self-blame attributions among rape survivors are often influenced by myths about rape that are commonly held in society, which tend to blame rape victims for being assaulted.[31] One comparative study found that South Africans are more likely than Australians to blame rape survivors.[32] Such attitudes are likely to be an important influence in the development of self-blame beliefs among South African rape survivors. However, survivors of other kinds of trauma also often blame themselves when trying to find an explanation for the trauma. People who have been the victim of a violent crime sometimes feel that the assault would not have happened if they had done certain things differently, such as taking more precautions and protective measures (for example, avoiding certain areas, not driving alone, locking their car doors or being more vigilant and aware of what was going on around them).[33] People who have received a cancer diagnosis may attribute the illness to past eating behaviours or other lifestyle factors.[34] Behavioural self-blame allows the survivor to regain some sense of personal control over events, because they identify behaviours that could be changed in order to minimise the chances of experiencing a similar trauma in the future.[35] This maintains a belief in a controllable world, where specific behaviours result in specific outcomes.

Another type of self-blame used by trauma survivors to explain why the trauma happened to them is characterological self-blame.[36] Here the survivor focuses blame on their own character or personal qualities – they come to believe that 'the trauma happened to me because of who I *am*' not 'because of what I did or did not *do*'. For example, someone who has been the victim of a violent crime might believe that 'the criminal chose me because he can see I'm weak' or 'this happened because I attract disaster', while a rape survivor may believe that the rape happened because 'I'm too trusting' or 'I'm such a poor judge of character'. The tendency towards characterological self-blame after a trauma is influenced by the person's schemas or beliefs about themselves prior to the trauma, which are in turn influenced by early relationships (such as with parents) that impact on self-esteem and self-worth, and by previous experiences of trauma. Thus, people who have survived early childhood abuse at the hands of a parent or other caretaker may be particularly likely to engage in characterological self-blame, as they struggle to make sense of why someone who is supposed to love and care for them would hurt them.[37] Sometimes, the only way to make sense of this is for the child to believe that he or she somehow deserved the abuse, for example because 'I am a bad person and deserve to be punished', or 'there is something wrong with me as a person'. Children are particularly prone to self-blame because, developmentally, they are egocentric in their understanding of the world; but these feelings of innate badness and shame, related to a sense that they somehow invited or deserved the abuse, often persist into adulthood.

Earlier research suggested that trauma survivors tend to engage in either one or the other form of self-blame after a trauma, and that behavioural self-blame is related to better adjustment after trauma than characterological self-blame, as the former is associated with a sense of future control over events (our behaviour can usually be changed), while the latter creates a sense of being a chronic or perpetual victim.[38] However, more recent research with rape survivors[39] and with women newly diagnosed with breast cancer[40] found that participants engaged in both types of self-blame simultaneously and that both types were associated with high distress levels after trauma. While behavioural self-blame can increase one's sense of control over the world, it can also increase feelings of distress and incompetence after a trauma. Clinicians working with rape survivors in the United States have found that behavioural self-blame, such as berating oneself for freezing during the rape or for not fighting back hard enough, reinforce feelings of incompetence and shame.[41] More locally, clinicians working with the mothers of children who have sustained serious burn injuries in informal dwellings in Cape Town have found that these parents struggle with feelings of self-blame for not preventing the accident, or for not treating the burn injury properly. This results in extreme distress and powerful feelings of guilt, especially if others in the family or community also blame the parent's behaviour for the child's injury.[42] As with rape survivors, societal attitudes of blame seem to powerfully influence the explanatory strategies that these parents develop in order to make meaning of the trauma of a child's burn injury. In general it seems that self-recrimination or self-blame of whatever kind is counterproductive to trauma recovery and is often associated with elevated depressive symptoms and lower self-esteem.

Redefining the event and its impact

Another way in which trauma survivors try to make sense of the event and its impact is by redefining the event to minimise the degree to which it disrupts the survivor's existing assumptive framework.[43] One common way of doing this is by minimising the perceived impact of the event by comparing oneself with others who have had a worse experience (a process called 'downward comparison'). Often after a trauma such as a hijacking or an armed assault, other people will tell the survivor 'you're so lucky it wasn't worse; you could have been killed!'. Sometimes, this response from others can feel very invalidating and judgmental for the survivor, who feels that they are not supposed to feel so distressed in response to a relatively 'minor' assault. However, many survivors of trauma may themselves use such comparison processes as a means of retaining a sense of a benevolent world that has in some way protected them from a worse outcome. For example, survivors of interpersonal assaults or accidents may compare themselves with others who have had a similar experience but who have suffered greater physical injury, and survivors of a natural disaster who have lost many of their material possessions may compare themselves with others who have lost even more.[44] The study conducted with crime survivors in Cape Town found that several participants felt themselves lucky after making comparisons to hypothetical worse outcomes (such as being killed or being threatened with a gun instead of with a knife), and that this helped to rebuild their assumptions about the benevolence of the world and to reassure them with regard to their needs for safety and control.[45]

Another form of comparison that survivors may use to redefine the impact of the event is to compare their coping with that of others.[46] Thus survivors might come to believe that they are coping well compared to how others might cope under the same circumstances. Although we have seen in the previous chapter that most trauma survivors actually return to normal functioning fairly quickly, comparison to others who would be coping less well can help the survivor to feel competent and capable in the aftermath of a trauma. On the other hand, some survivors compare themselves unfavourably with the perceived norm, feeling that they are coping worse than other people would after a similar experience. This may leave the survivor feeling increasingly incompetent, vulnerable and ashamed of their inability to 'rise above' the trauma.

Beyond Comprehensibility: The Search For Significance

Trauma can have an impact on our belief and meaning systems that goes beyond trying to develop an explanation for why the trauma happened. For some survivors, meaning-making after trauma may also involve a consideration of the possible lessons and benefits of having survived an extremely stressful event. Research indicates that many, although by no means all, trauma survivors spontaneously (that is, without the assistance of counselling or therapy) identify positive outcomes from their trauma experience. Interestingly, it appears that this process often occurs in parallel with the negative psychological impact of trauma – that is, trauma survivors can experience PTSD and other psychiatric symptoms after trauma while also experiencing some positive outcomes from the experience. Research findings on the positive outcomes of trauma, and on their relationship with the negative outcomes, will be discussed in this section.

Finding value and purpose in adversity

Although writings about the struggle to find value in suffering have historically been the domain of philosophy and theology, in more recent times this concept has been explored in the psychological literature on trauma. The psychiatrist Viktor Frankl's[47] account of his concentration camp experiences, and his theory of logotherapy (from the Greek word for both *meaning* and *spirit*), is perhaps the earliest psychological text that specifically explores the question of finding value in deeply traumatic experiences. He argued that the search for meaning in life is a primary motivational force for human beings, and that, even when one is trapped in a situation of unavoidable suffering, small but meaningful goals can be developed – such as finding ways to engage in ethical or 'right' conduct when other people are not. Much more recently, several research studies have documented a range of meaningful outcomes that survivors of many different kinds of trauma have identified as a result of their experience of adversity. The identification of meaningful outcomes is usually a long-term process – it can seldom be achieved in the immediate aftermath of a trauma and is more likely to emerge after many months or even years of internal processing and reflection.[48]

The first possible type of meaningful outcome that may be experienced after a trauma is positive changes in perceptions of the self.[49] This generally entails an enhanced sense of personal strength and competence as a result of having survived something very difficult. Survivors are often surprised by the resilience and reserves of strength that they are able to draw on from deep inside themselves in order to cope with a trauma. But positive perceptions of the self after trauma can also involve developing a greater respect for one's vulnerabilities. Survivors of many different types of trauma have reported that the trauma experience was so emotionally devastating that it forced them to change longstanding coping patterns of denying their feelings of vulnerability or distress and of avoiding asking other people for help. While this was difficult and even shameful to do at the time, ultimately it allowed them to gain more knowledge and acceptance of their vulnerabilities and of the value of being able to depend on others for support in times of distress.

A second area of meaningful outcomes commonly reported by trauma survivors is improvements in relationships with others.[50] Firstly, survivors have reported that, as a result of having to depend on others for emotional support in order to cope with the trauma, they have developed a greater capacity for emotional expressiveness and for disclosing their feelings and fears to others. This has resulted in a deeper sense of trust and greater interpersonal intimacy with important people in their lives. Secondly, trauma survivors often emerge from the experience with increased compassion and empathy for others. While survivors may have previously been able to intellectually understand and sympathise with the suffering of others, their personal experience of trauma allows for a richer emotional insight into the pain and distress of other people, and the emergence of a deeper capacity for compassion towards others. Finally, improved relationships with others after the trauma often evolve through the survivor becoming involved in altruistic social causes that provide them with a feeling of connection to others and with a greater sense of value and purpose through making a contribution to others. For example, many survivors report becoming involved in activities that feel constructive for them, such as fundraising for a trauma organisation, training to be a trauma counsellor or volunteering as a police reservist.

Another area of meaning that can arise after a trauma is a changed philosophy of life.[51] This includes a greater appreciation of small things that were previously taken for granted – for example, loving moments with one's family, a beautiful sunset, the kindness of other people. Whether a traumatic experience involves a deliberate assault by another person, actual or near physical injury due to an accident or natural disaster or the diagnosis of a life-threatening illness, being faced with one's own mortality and with the threat of losing everything can sometimes serve to highlight the joy and beauty that is inherent in the simplest of things. A changed philosophy of life after a trauma can therefore also result in a re-ordering of priorities, including decisions to spend less time and emotional energy on work and more on family and other relationships, and to devote time and energy to helping others rather than to achieving one's own goals. Finally, a changed philosophy of life can also entail the development of new or stronger spiritual or existential beliefs that add a richer dimension of meaning and purpose to the survivor's life.

The majority of the research on the positive outcomes of trauma has been conducted in socio-economically developed countries such as the United States and Canada. However, in some exploratory studies South African survivors of different forms of trauma have also identified a number of post-trauma benefits. Using the Post Traumatic Growth Inventory (PTGI), a study of sixty-seven parents who had experienced the loss of a child found evidence that both mothers and fathers perceived some benefits from their experiences of loss, and that the perception of benefits increased with the passing of time since the bereavement.[52] A set of semi-structured interviews with small groups of violent crime survivors, rape survivors and mothers who had lost a child to cancer explored whether these three groups perceived any benefit or value emerging from their traumatic experiences, without suggesting to participants what these benefits might be. The interviews were conducted several months or years after the participants had experienced the trauma about which they were being interviewed, in order to allow time for post-trauma meaning-making to occur. The participants were from a range of different language and cultural groups. Although not all survivors identified post-trauma benefits, the majority of them did. The interviews yielded remarkably similar themes of positive meaning-making after trauma across these groups, and these themes replicated those reported in international studies.[53] See Table 4.1 for a summary of the post-trauma benefits reported across these three groups. In a larger-scale study comparing scores on the PTGI across 135 survivors of various types of trauma (including chronic illness, traumatic bereavement, crime, and accident or injury), 76 per cent of the sample reported moderate or high posttraumatic growth, with survivors of a traumatic bereavement reporting the greatest amount of growth and survivors of crime reporting the lowest.[54] These findings suggest that South Africans who have survived a variety of potentially traumatic events are often, though by no means always, able to identify some value or benefit arising from their experience.

The findings of international and local research therefore seem to indicate that many trauma survivors use the trauma as an opportunity to re-evaluate their lives in a more positive way, and that positive transformation after trauma represents not simply a return to normal or baseline functioning, but rather may entail the achievement of a higher level of fulfilment than existed before the trauma.[55] Positive outcomes after trauma have thus often been termed 'posttraumatic growth'.[56] But how can growth occur in response to extreme adversity? As discussed above, a severe trauma, and the threatened losses that accompany it, throws into stark contrast previously unrecognised or unappreciated aspects of the survivor's daily life, allowing these to be 'seen' and appreciated for the first time. In addition, in order to cope with the trauma, the survivor often has to draw on internal and external resources that they have simply not had to access previously. These resources also become 'seen' and appreciated for the first time. Finally, since the trauma often does not seem to fit with the existing

Table 4.1

Post-trauma benefits reported by participants in a study comparing three groups of South African trauma survivors

	Rape survivors (n = 10)	Survivors of violent crime (n = 10)	Mothers who have lost a child to cancer (n = 10)
Greater compassion for others	*		*
More meaningful relationships with others	*	*	*
Engaging in altruistic activities to help others	*		*
Greater appreciation of 'little things' in life		*	*
Feeling emotionally stronger	*	*	*

Source: Kaminer, Booley, Lipshitz & Thacker, 2009

beliefs and expectations held by the trauma survivor, these beliefs and expectations need to be re-examined. A traumatic event can therefore be conceptualised as a turning point, watershed, crossroad or choice-point in the survivor's life in which previous values, priorities and ways of being can be re-considered, and a change in the 'plot' of the survivor's life-narrative towards a more purposeful and significant one becomes possible.[57] Some authors have suggested that, in this way, the trauma can be 'honoured' as an opportunity for growth, at the same time as recognising the losses that the trauma has brought.[58]

A danger of this literature on the potential benefits of trauma is that trauma survivors who are not able to identify any benefits from their trauma experience may feel that they are somehow deficient. Especially when our popular culture emphasises the importance of using positive thinking to overcome adversity, it is all too easy to conclude that trauma survivors *should* be able to find some value in their suffering. However, while many survivors do identify some positive outcomes of their trauma experience as time goes on, many other survivors do not. They continue to struggle with a sense of emptiness and meaningless. The search for meaning after trauma is a deeply personal process and there is no 'right' way to engage in, or resolve, this difficult and often painful journey. Furthermore, the development of posttraumatic growth implies some sort of *post*-traumatic space or phase during which the survivor can reflect on the meaning of the trauma experience. In a context of continuous traumatisation, such as living in a situation of ongoing community and/or domestic violence, the survivor may never have such a space. They may feel perpetually in fear of danger, or may shut themselves down emotionally in order to cope – emotional states that do not allow for internal reflection. Studies of benefit-finding have not yet been conducted with South Africans living in conditions of continuous violence and trauma. An additional caution, as we shall see in the next section, is that there is no clear and direct relationship between finding positive outcomes after trauma and actual psychological recovery from trauma.

The relationship between positive and negative outcomes of trauma

It seems logical that being able to find positive outcomes in the aftermath of a traumatic experience would assist a trauma survivor to recover from their experience and regain a state of psychological wellness. However, this does not necessarily appear to be the case. Within the research on the psychological outcomes of trauma, there is no consistent trend in the relationship between posttraumatic growth (that is, finding benefit or value in a trauma experience) and psychological well-being.[59] Many studies have found that posttraumatic growth is related to lower levels of psychological distress – that is, trauma survivors who report posttraumatic growth also report less psychological distress than survivors who do not report posttraumatic growth. However, it is not clear whether finding benefits in the trauma experience results in a decrease in psychological distress, whether a decrease in psychological distress makes it possible to begin identifying value in the trauma experience or whether there is no direct causal relationship between the two dimensions of experience. A few studies have reported no relationship at all between posttraumatic growth and psychological distress, while some other studies have found that identifying benefits of a trauma experience is, in fact, associated with an increase in psychological distress, an increase in intrusive and avoidance symptoms of PTSD, and worse subjective physical health – in other words, people who report posttraumatic growth also sometimes report worse psychological outcomes than people who do not report posttraumatic growth.[60]

While some of the variation in research findings may be the result of different methodologies used across studies (for example, posttraumatic growth has been conceptualised and measured in different ways by different researchers, and the populations of trauma survivors that have been sampled in these studies differ along a number of variables), several other explanations have been suggested for the finding that posttraumatic growth is not always associated with improved psychological well-being. Firstly, it is possible that posttraumatic distress and posttraumatic growth are separate, but parallel, processes or dimensions[61] – that is, in the aftermath of trauma, psychological growth experiences do not put an end to distress. They simply occur in parallel with distress. Secondly, it is possible that psychological distress is necessary in order for meaning-making to occur.[62] Struggling with intrusive reminders of the trauma and experiencing some degree of subjective emotional pain may provide the impetus for ruminating about the meaning of the trauma, for trying to make sense of it. Psychological growth occurs in the aftermath of emotional upheaval, precipitated by a psychologically seismic event;[63] if a trauma has little emotional impact, there is no need to try to understand the meaning of the trauma. Interestingly, some studies have found that posttraumatic growth is more likely to occur when there are moderate levels of PTSD, rather than mild or severe symptoms[64] – mild symptoms may not create enough impetus to engage in meaning-making strategies such as benefit-finding, while severe symptoms may prevent any reflective processing of the traumatic event. Thirdly, it has been argued that there may be a self-deceptive, illusory aspect to posttraumatic growth.[65] When faced with feelings of vulnerability after a trauma, survivors may respond with positive but slightly distorted beliefs about themselves and the future. This is a form of cognitive avoidance or denial of the difficulties that the trauma represents, which may occur temporarily as a short-term coping strategy in the immediate aftermath of the trauma and which may be replaced by more authentic posttraumatic growth (or not) over the long term. Together, these theories may account for the apparently contradictory findings across studies regarding the relationship between negative and positive outcomes of trauma.

Conclusion

An important psychological consequence of trauma is a struggle to make meaning of the event. After an experience of trauma, the survivor's world can never be quite the same again. Previous beliefs and assumptions may be profoundly challenged and the survivor must search for new beliefs and assumptions that can enable him or her to make sense of what has taken place and to go forward into the future. For some survivors, the trauma may leave behind an ongoing sense of meaninglessness, raising troubling questions about themselves, others and the world for which no satisfactory answer can be found. Others may develop a new appreciation for themselves, other people and life in general. Yet others may experience a combination of feelings – it seems that the outcomes of trauma are not purely negative or positive, but often a complex mix of the two. Regardless of the outcome, the process of struggling to answer the question 'why?' is an important part of trying to adapt to a traumatic experience.

Chapter 5

TRAUMA INTERVENTIONS FOR INDIVIDUALS, GROUPS AND COMMUNITIES

Having spent considerable time exploring the prevalence of trauma in society in general and in South Africa in particular, as well as the impact of trauma in terms of both symptoms and alterations to meaning, it is important to look at what can be done to address these effects. The discussion of interventions will include a focus on psychotherapeutic and alternative, community-based interventions as well as a brief section on pharmacotherapy or drug treatment. The chapter will also address interventions as they are formulated to assist individuals, groups and communities.

Dealing with the impact of traumatic events has long been the focus of psychotherapists, with Freud's early work in the 1800s as a prime example. However, with the formalisation and refinement of the diagnosis of Acute Stress Disorder(ASD) and PTSD, over the last ten to twenty years there has been renewed interest in treatment approaches for trauma, and a move to more research-based practice. There is a large array of therapeutic approaches to dealing with traumatic stress with considerable debate about the merits and demerits of various models of intervention. In addition to the more conventional 'talking-based' types of therapy and counselling, there are also more creative and body-oriented interventions. It is also not uncommon for psychotropic medication to be prescribed for trauma clients alongside psychotherapy. As will be discussed further in Chapter 6, play therapy is also commonly used to assist traumatised children to process traumatic events.

Over and above professional counselling and psychotherapeutic treatments that might be individual- or group-focused, the impact of traumatic events has also been recognised as significant by social and community groups. In many instances members of a particular geographical or value-based community have been known to spontaneously generate rituals and practices to mark and heal the impact of trauma, recognising that in addition to having individual effects, trauma damages interpersonal bonds and tests community cohesion. In some cases members of society, previously unknown to each other, who have undergone a similar traumatic experience have also developed mechanisms for sharing and support that transcend group psychotherapy. Such kinds of community-based initiatives have been particularly important in South Africa where professional services are not always easily available and accessible and where communal aspects of identity have been strongly inculcated in traditional African culture and belief systems.

This chapter will first discuss more individually oriented and formally based interventions before addressing more community-focused interventions.

Individual Psychotherapy and Counselling

The context

In a seminal work in the traumatic stress field, Judith Herman[1] suggests that there are three crucial aspects to all treatment of traumatic stress. Firstly, it is necessary to establish a sense of safety for the individual; secondly, it is important to process and integrate the trauma in some way, and thirdly, it is important for some kind of re-engagement with the larger community to be facilitated. She asserts that if the first of these elements is not in place it is virtually impossible for the other aspects of trauma work to be initiated and to be successful. It makes sense that a person who feels unsafe in reality in the present is unlikely to be able to engage in a therapy process that involves processing traumatic material, since this inevitably evokes strong anxiety. In a situation of experienced danger it would be irresponsible to add to current anxiety and to possibly tamper with the psychological defences a person has in place in order to deal with ongoing threats. This may be the case for people living in the conditions of 'continuous traumatic stress' described in Chapter 3. This issue will be returned to further, but at this point it is important to emphasise that, as far as possible, trauma therapy assumes that a client's safety has been secured prior to other aspects of intervention.

A further dimension influencing choices about intervention is the immediacy of the traumatising event and the severity of the diagnostic symptom picture. A person who comes for therapy twenty-four hours after a rape will present differently from someone who decides to seek therapy three years after the rape event. Until recently it was assumed that trauma counselling should be offered as soon as possible after the trauma, within seventy-two hours if at all possible. However, based on mixed reports and some critical research findings that will be discussed under the section on debriefing, it is now generally thought that early support is important but that optimal therapeutic work may only be possible some time after the trauma, once the initial shock and disorganisation has passed.[2] Although people may sometimes need to be encouraged to seek counselling, given a tendency to want to avoid trauma associations, it is very important that they feel a sense of choice in engaging in counselling. This is significant in light of the fact that trauma involves loss of control and helplessness. There are also different treatment implications depending upon whether a person is diagnosable as suffering from ASD, or Acute, Chronic or Delayed-onset forms of PTSD. Generally the longer a person has been symptomatic, the deeper and longer therapy will need to be, although there are exceptions to this. Chronic forms of PTSD are particularly difficult to treat and may require multiple forms of intervention including medication, individual, couple and family therapy, as well as social support.

A useful way of thinking about trauma counselling is to divide it into three different sub-fields: acute interventions or debriefing, short-term counselling, and long-term counselling or psychotherapy. Generally ASD is treated by means of debriefing or short-term counselling, whereas PTSD is treated by means of short-term or long-term psychotherapy.

At Camden Trauma Clinic in London a useful distinction has been made between what staff broadly term 'simple' and complex' forms of trauma, the latter involving some sort of deliberate degradation or humiliation of the victim. Their Cognitive Behavioural Therapy (CBT)-based treatment protocol entails an eight-session intervention for 'simple' trauma cases and a twenty-session intervention for 'complex' cases.

Trauma practitioners usually select one of the three therapeutic forms available (acute, short-term or long-term) based on a number of different situational and organisational criteria. In South Africa, a significant element in determining intervention, beyond severity of traumatisation and length of time elapsed since the event, is whether survivors can easily access services. Working-class clients, such as security guards and domestic workers, may find it difficult to take time off work and services may be geographically distant and transport too expensive. Thus although longer-term work might be desirable in some cases, brief-term work is often all that is feasible and therapeutic modalities need to be tailored to this limitation. However, before looking further at contextually specific South African issues in treatment, it is important to discuss what each of the three broad treatment types encompasses.

Acute or 'frontline' interventions

Acute interventions are often subsumed under the term 'trauma debriefing' but include more extensive approaches than this. Raphael and Dobson[3] include emergency interventions, psychological first aid, military interventions and crisis intervention, together with debriefing, as all constituting 'acute' interventions. They argue that while acute trauma interventions have been defined in terms of their almost immediate use after damaging events, 'the provision of trauma counselling may take place in the early days or even weeks and can still be considered acute',[4] in part based on the fact that full-blown PTSD has not developed.

The term 'debriefing' was originally associated with military and paramilitary procedures and in this context referred to the sharing of information after a particular exercise or manoeuvre in an attempt to resolve issues for participants. The use of the term within the trauma field became popular in the 1970s and 'debriefing' has become part of everyday discourse concerning trauma treatment. It is also within the military that the emphasis on intervention soon after an incident has been emphasised. For example, the acronym for trauma intervention that is used in the Israeli military, which influenced previous South African National Defence Force (SANDF) thinking, is PIE, standing for Proximity, Immediacy and Expectancy. The idea behind this approach is that troops in action should be treated close to the battle front, as quickly as possible, with the expectation that they return to active combat within a relatively short period of time. This intervention was designed to assist the military institution but it was also hoped that it would ameliorate the development of more serious combat trauma. While the approach seems to have been successful in getting soldiers to return to active combat, the long-term effects have not been well researched and it is not clear that this prevented the later development of PTSD. In fact, it is possible that the intervention led to increased vulnerability to pathology later: 'whether keeping people functional but in so doing keeping them in a situation where they may be traumatised again (and again) is ultimately helpful to outcomes is a critical question for future research'.[5] This question still has bearing in broader terms for various groups in contemporary society; for example, for men working in the South African security industry, many of whom are ex-soldiers. Those involved in the cash transportation business, for instance, face daily danger and witness colleagues injured and murdered. Debriefing for such personnel has to take account of the fact that many of these men have no choice but to return to the same working conditions within days of life-threatening incidents.

Historically it is interesting to observe that while some psychological debriefing along the lines discussed was used in the South African Defence Force (SADF) in the later stages of the war fought in Angola and Namibia, traumatic stress in war veterans within the country amongst both SADF and liberation fighters has generally gone untreated in the period following demobilisation and return to civilian life. Although there are a number of organisations dealing with the current difficulties of ex-combatants, trauma treatment is still often scanty and difficult to implement because of the lapse of time since combat-related trauma exposure and the preoccupation with pressing current social problems, such as unemployment. In this respect, trauma treatment facilities for South African veterans have been under-developed relative to those offered to veterans in the United States, the population who, in many respects, put posttraumatic stress disorder and its treatment on the world map. One local intervention with ex-combatants from both formal and informal military structures has been what is generally termed 'Wilderness Therapy' and will be discussed later under the section on group intervention, since it is not an acute form of intervention.

Returning to the discussion of debriefing, the approach to intervention known as debriefing is generally synonymous with what more accurately is called Critical Incident Stress Debriefing (CISD). CISD was initially developed by Mitchell[6] to address the psychological effects of work stress in emergency service workers, such as paramedics and fire fighters. It was designed as a group intervention to be used within seventy-two hours of a particular incident and was intended to allow for discharge of distress or the dilution of the possible 'toxic' effects of intervening in traumatic situations, aimed in turn at the prevention of later PTSD. For example, debriefing was used with fire fighters who were involved in removing children's bodies from the scene of the Oklahoma bombing with the expectation that this would reduce later psychological distress. Dyregov's[7] group model of intervention known as Psychological Debriefing (PD), also designed for use with 'helpers', is the other prominent debriefing model and is sometimes used in conjunction with the Mitchell model. Neither CISD nor PD appear to be used routinely with emergency service workers in South Africa, but debriefing may be employed in organisations after particularly horrific incidents, and involve both group and individual debriefing.

CISD involves seven set steps of intervention and may be conducted in groups as large as ten to twenty people.[8] The seven components are: introduction, expectations and facts, thoughts and impressions, emotional reactions, normalisation, future planning and coping, and disengagement.[9] The model involves reflecting back upon and recounting various aspects of the traumatic incident in a deliberately structured manner, for example, separating out thoughts about the event in one re-telling from a re-telling focused on the more emotional aspects. It is possible that this allows for manageable engagement with difficult content, or what Horowitz[10] refers to as 'optimal dosing'. In addition the intervention has a strong psychoeducational component. Dyregov's PD[11] has many similar elements but deals with the trauma story in a less tightly compartmentalised way and places more weight on stimulating group processes, such as the provision of peer support. A summary of the common elements of most debriefings is as follows:

> During a PD, participants are encouraged to provide a full narrative account of the trauma that encompasses facts, cognitions, and feelings. In addition, emotional reactions to the trauma are considered in some detail with the emphasis on normalisation. Individuals are reassured that they are responding normally to an abnormal event, are prepared for later emotional reactions and told how to deal with them and where to find further support if necessary.[12]

Following the introduction of PD into the trauma field in the 1980s this kind of intervention became used in increasingly wider settings. PD became the treatment of choice not only for groups, but also for individuals, and for both direct and indirect victims of traumatic events. For example, PD has been used after natural disasters, motor vehicle accidents (MVAs) and violent crime incidents, amongst others. In South Africa, PD and CISD have been widely used in the banking and retail industry to assist staff after armed robberies and work-place incidents (such as suicides), and have been provided mostly by Employee Assistance (EA) personnel. Psychologists are also commonly called in to debrief families who have been through trauma or members of organisations in which traumatic incidents have taken place, including schools. For example, following the suicide of a work colleague or fellow pupil, debriefers may be called in to address the fall-out in an organisation or school, often attempting to assess the likelihood of later symptom development amongst members of the group as part of their task. More recently there has been increasing concern amongst trauma specialists that debriefing has become over-used, sometimes in contexts that are inappropriate and sometimes by inexperienced practitioners. This is in part because it has become a fairly lucrative practice, particularly for counsellors servicing large organisations. While the moral imperative to help people who have been traumatised in their workplace is understandable, the use of debriefing is sometimes rather formulaic and other interventions, such as improving working conditions or advising management about how best to offer support to their staff, might be more appropriate. Despite the fact that assessment of risk for the development of pathology is usually intrinsic in debriefing, organisations are not always willing to fund recommended follow-up services. The popularity of debriefing as a trauma intervention is not peculiar to South Africa and in the late 1990s researchers from the United Kingdom began to review the widespread use of debriefing and to question its efficacy.

In their meta-theoretical study of the results of a range of research studies into the efficacy of trauma debriefing, Rose and Bisson[13] established that the grounds for the continued use of CISD and other forms of debriefing were rather shaky. Of the six reasonably controlled studies of treatment that they were able to identify and review, there was evidence of minor improvement in two studies, of no improvement in another two studies and, in the remaining two studies, some suggestion that debriefing might even be detrimental in terms of creating a vulnerability to later pathology. It is possible that debriefing offered too early may 're-traumatise' individuals in that it exposes them to emotionally arousing subject matter at a point at which it might be more beneficial for natural defences to operate to allow for more gradual habituation to the material. It has also been suggested that group debriefing may expose members to new traumatic material as details of different people's experience during the trauma are recounted, also possibly leading to increased traumatisation. Despite the lack of clear evidence for the efficacy of psychological debriefing it is worth noting that where participant evaluations of their experiences of the debriefing were sought, in the vast majority of cases survivors themselves perceived the intervention as beneficial.[14] It is now generally accepted that, while some sort of frontline support is useful to individuals immediately following a trauma because it provides some emotional containment and structure (what some have called 'tea and sympathy'), any thorough processing of the event may be better introduced some time after the event when people are less disorientated, disorganised and vulnerable. However, the importance of perceived support should not be under-estimated and it may be that intervention of a supportive kind soon after the occurrence of a trauma is particularly important in helping to counteract people's experience of other people as harmful and in making people aware of the fact that further assistance can be sought. It seems that debriefing might have its place if introduced thoughtfully in a considered, rather than automatic 'one size fits all' kind of way. Practitioners have begun to look at the merits of 'Emergency Support' or 'Psychological First Aid' rather than necessarily offering debriefing in the form associated with CISD.

Short- and medium-term counselling
The most common and widely used forms of intervention in the trauma field would fall into the category of brief- to medium-term intervention, with therapy lasting anything from two sessions to several months. Structured approaches may, for example, involve a set of either four to six, or alternatively eight to twelve sessions. Such counselling is aimed at those suffering from ASD, PTSD or other related trauma conditions. There are a range of different types or models of what is generally referred to as 'short-term' counselling interventions, including models based in mainstream paradigms of psychotherapy, such as cognitive behaviour therapy (CBT) and psychodynamic therapy, as well as Eye Movement Desensitisation and Reprocessing (EMDR) and other approaches that are sometimes collectively referred to as the 'power' or 'neoteric' or new therapies. The use of pharmacotherapy will be discussed somewhat later as it straddles both short- and long-term trauma intervention.

Mainstream approaches
The more mainstream approaches to short-term treatment of traumatic stress include cognitive behaviour therapy, narrative therapy, psychodynamic therapy and integrative therapeutic approaches.

Cognitive Behaviour Therapy

Cognitive behavioural treatments for traumatic stress share in common that they are based on an understanding of symptoms as stemming from maladaptive learning and conditioning that takes place in response to traumatic stimuli. There are many different treatment protocols and types that fall under the umbrella of CBT treatment, including Foa and colleagues' Prolonged Exposure (PE),[15] Resick and Schnicke's Cognitive Processing Therapy (CPT),[16] Meichenbaum's Stress Inoculation Training (SIT)[17] and Ehler's and Clark's Cognitive Therapy (CT).[18] These types of CBT treatment are usually prescriptive, detailed well into manuals and take between nine to sixteen sessions to implement. Different aspects may be used in combination at times. Generally, at least three different principles are involved in CBT treatment of trauma, namely repeated exposure to traumatic memories and traumatic reminders in order to reduce the anxiety associated with these and habituate the client to such material; developing strategies to manage anxiety, such as relaxation training or thought-stopping; and cognitive restructuring in order to modify any maladaptive beliefs that may have developed in relation to the trauma (such as those already discussed in Chapter 4).

Foa and colleagues' approach requires not only that the client recount the trauma repeatedly in therapy, but that the sessions are recorded and then played back to the client between consultations.[19] The therapy is based within a classical conditioning framework which holds that the process of traumatisation entails the association of previously neutral stimuli with anxiety and fear and that this pairing is followed by consequent avoidance of reminders of the event. For example, a woman who had been raped by a man wearing a green overall became agitated whenever she encountered a man wearing green and would move as far away from him as possible. The avoidance of feared objects, situations and people means that new learning cannot take place and the cycle of association is reinforced. Exposure to traumatic material in the supportive context of the therapeutic relationship is designed to reduce the connection between trauma memories and high levels of fear and arousal, while gradual exposure to realistically unthreatening traumatic reminders outside of the therapy room aims to modify the survivor's cycle of avoidance. This approach appears to have considerable benefit if the survivor can tolerate the treatment, which entails willingness to manage high levels of anxiety. Resick and Schicke's CPT also involves exposure elements, including the writing of a personal account of what happened, but places greater weight on working with the maladaptive thoughts that are generated by the trauma.[20] For example, over-generalisation, self-recrimination and negativity about the future would all be tackled using forms of cognitive restructuring. Meichenbaum's SIT is designed to look at managing future anxiety, amongst other aspects, and helps the person to imagine approaching feared situations and coping with these.[21] Role-plays with the therapist and strategies for gradually approaching feared, but realistically safe, situations may be used to help the survivor to regain control. For example, someone who fears driving after an accident might be encouraged just to sit in a car initially, then to be a passenger, then to drive a short distance in a safe setting, then to drive further and so on. In addition to most of the aspects of treatment already described, Ehlers et al's CT requires that the client specifically revisit what they refer to as the 'hotspots' (or the most distressing and anxiety-provoking aspects) within the trauma experience so as to examine the associations to these emotionally charged elements and detoxify them.[22] There is also attention to modifying excessively negative appraisals of the event and its consequences.

CBT approaches generally employ a strong psychoeducational component and the client is usually informed about the impact of traumatic stressors and the reasoning behind treatment. Although there are some differences among CBT approaches, in general CBT has the clearest proven efficacy in treating trauma and is probably the treatment of choice of most practitioners.[23] However, it is important to point out that protocol-based CBT therapy is often difficult to implement in South Africa, in part because of a lack of trained professionals and in part because clients may find it difficult to attend structured counselling for the requisite number of sessions. Language and other resource barriers also preclude the easy replication of international models and it is often the case that aspects of CBT-based approaches are used rather than entire protocols. From a research perspective, perhaps because the procedures used in CBT are easier to replicate, since they are based in many instances on set protocols, CBT approaches have tended to be more concertedly researched than psychodynamic, narrative and integrative approaches.

Narrative therapy

Although not as widely documented and used in the treatment of trauma as either CBT or psychodynamic approaches, narrative therapy has also been employed to assist traumatised clients. Since narrative therapy is focused on re-authoring people's life stories and altering meaning in a way that benefits the client and increases his/her sense of personal agency or potency, it makes sense that this is an approach that has been used to deal with trauma. The narrative therapy literature proposes that adverse or traumatic experiences can become the basis for stories of resilience and survival and that these aspects of the story can be thickened and enriched.[24] In narrative therapy, 'the stories can be separated from the survivor. Rather than emphasising that the client has been the victim of a traumatic event, the client can almost immediately be seen as a survivor who wants to move forward from the traumatic experience. In addition, the therapy encourages that power be collaborative rather than enforced over the client, a basic rule in trauma treatment'.[25] Narrative therapy has been successfully used with African and Asian refugee populations with the suggestion that such an approach may be compatible with traditional oral story telling practices.[26] In addition, in his more recent writings Meichenbaum has incorporated aspects of narrative theory into his trauma treatment approach, referring to it as 'narrative constructivist'.[27] Meichenbaum encourages therapists to work collaboratively with the client to reconstruct the traumatic event/s in such a way that the survivor is able to integrate and live with his or her interpretation and version of what happened. This aspect of therapeutic work resonates with the second central element of trauma work outlined by Herman as discussed at the outset of this chapter.

The narrative approach also underpins a more politically oriented approach to trauma treatment known as testimony therapy.[28] In testimony therapy, the client is assisted to tell and document the story of their traumatisation or tribulation in such a way that the telling represents a formal record of the event. This record or testimony may be explicitly intended to become part of the public record with the aim of influencing policy or providing a basis for lobbying, prosecution or restitution. This approach has been used primarily with victims of political repression, torture or violence.[29] In addition to serving a personal function, the telling and detailed documentation of the story may serve an empowering function in providing the survivor with some validation and potential agency. Since most repression and torture takes place in hidden and intimidating circumstances, there is an element of defiance or resistance in testimony therapy. Clearly clients exercise choice in how material is documented and where their stories are stored and appear. Currently, for example, a number of torture survivors from a neighbouring African country have provided accounts of their experiences as part of their treatment in order to contribute to a dossier of evidence on torture that may be used to exert political pressure on those employing such methods of control. Other refugee groups in South Africa have also extended narrative aspects of their therapy into 'testimony' in order to expose atrocities committed in their countries of origin and to appeal to the collective South African conscience in terms of their experiences of being treated as illegitimate in the country. The idea that giving public testimony at the Truth and Reconciliation Commission of South Africa would be beneficial (or even therapeutic) to victims and their families, also had its origins in this kind of testimony approach to trauma and therapy. While existing evidence suggests that there were actually few psychological benefits of giving testimony to the TRC,[30] this is perhaps not surprising since TRC testimony did not occur within the context of a therapeutic relationship. Narrative therapy is thus an approach that has been modified for use in various contexts in South Africa, even if it is not widely documented as a trauma treatment model internationally.

Brief psychodynamic approaches
Although it is less usual for psychodynamic therapy to be offered on a short-term basis, there are specific forms of brief-term psychodynamic therapy. Brief Psychodynamic Psychotherapy (BPP) is a trauma-

focused form of therapy conducted over twelve to fifteen sessions.[31] In the trauma field short-term psychodynamic approaches to therapy have been associated primarily with the work of Horowitz[32] and Lindy[33] and tend to be located within the Ego-Psychology tradition. Horowitz's focal psychodynamic treatment focuses on assisting the client to assimilate the trauma material, based on an understanding that this 'information' has intruded in an overwhelming way and therefore cannot be processed according to usual psychic mechanisms. The work is supportive and strongly cognitive, rather than aimed at character change or emotional catharsis.[34] Clients are categorised in terms of whether they tend to be using an over-controlled or under-controlled defensive style in dealing with the trauma, associated respectively with whether they are manifesting more avoidant or more re-experiencing symptoms. Based on this, the therapist aims to assist the 'patient' to engage with the information associated with the trauma in a manageable way, by means of the 'optimal dosing' mentioned earlier, that is by helping the patient to 'divide the experience into suitably small and therefore potentially integrated units of information'.[35] The relational element of the therapy is emphasised in psychodynamic therapy for trauma, with the therapist aiming to provide a 'good object' experience that can gradually be internalised by the patient.

With trauma survivors, what is known in psychodynamic therapy as 'working through' consists of helping the client to make interpretive links between the trauma experience and other past and present aspects of their lives. The clinician 'helps the client understand the meaning of each unconscious process to achieve a balance between traumatic memories, external demands, and subjective needs'.[36] Or alternatively working through could be understood as, 'detailed conceptual, emotional, object-relations, and self-image implications of the traumatic stressor are addressed'.[37] It is clear that psychodynamic approaches to traumatic stress place a strong emphasis on the appreciation of the subjective meaning of the event for the individual and the linking of this to the person's 'internal world', while at the same time offering a supportive and containing relationship.

There has been little research into short-term psychodynamic treatment of trauma. However, one study on BPP established positive results in using this insight-oriented approach in the treatment of rape victims.[38] In another study comparing hypnotherapy, traumatic desensitisation and psychodynamic psychotherapy, the last mentioned approach proved more effective in reducing avoidance symptoms whereas the other two approaches were superior in diminishing re-experiencing symptoms.[39] In South Africa there is a fairly strong allegiance to psychodynamic and psychoanalytic psychotherapy amongst private psychotherapists and many of these practitioners treat trauma clients within this modality if they do take on trauma cases. Much of this work is long term rather than short term, however. In addition, there are some interesting traditions within British group psychoanalysis that have been applied in community work in South Africa, including in doing work with traumatised populations. Such applications tend to be more group focused. Given an interest in meaning-making amongst many South African trauma practitioners, perhaps because of the highly politicised nature of much trauma in the country, both historically and contemporarily, many draw on aspects of psychodynamic thinking in their work even if they work in more integrative or eclectic ways.

Integrative approaches
Although there is not a lot of literature on employing a specifically integrative approach to trauma intervention, in practice there is considerable evidence of integration within the field. This includes integration both across theoretical paradigms and across practical modalities of psychotherapy. For example, Horowitz's[40] information-processing approach is located within both a cognitive and a psycho-dynamic framework, Meichenbaum's[41] trauma approach encompasses both CBT and narrative approaches, and group and individual therapy may be used in conjunction in trauma work. Although most structured interventions are multimodal cognitive-behavioural packages, these are generally integrative in character since the historical sources of many specific techniques come from a range of therapy traditions.[42] Eagle has argued that there is a strong case to be made for integration in trauma work, given the interaction of external events with personality style and defensive patterns in producing trauma outcomes.[43] Thus

there is a need to address impact at different levels in different ways. Edwards concurs, arguing in a recent article on evidence-based practice for traumatic stress conditions, that the field has developed over time such that purist psychotherapeutic practitioners 'could be considered at the least narrow-minded and at most unethical since there is now abundant evidence that treatment needs to draw on a range of different interventions'.[44]

In Johannesburg, one of the commonly used local models of trauma intervention is known as the 'Wits Trauma Model', based on its development by a team of staff working at the University of the Witwatersrand (Wits). Drawing on a range of different existing frameworks and models for trauma intervention, including locally used rape trauma intervention models, the Wits approach is a short-term method for optimal use in two to twelve sessions with relatively straight-forward forms of trauma. However, it has been adapted for use with more complex forms of trauma such as traumatic bereavement and torture. The model is integrative as it draws upon both psychodynamic and cognitive-behavioural-theoretical underpinnings and consists of five components that can be used interchangeably in different sessions, depending on what the client brings to the sessions. In this respect, it is a flexible approach rather than a protocol-based intervention. The five components are: telling and retelling the story; normalisation of symptoms and responses (including fantasy elements, such as the fantasy of taking violent revenge against the perpetrator); addressing self-blame or survivor guilt (oriented towards the restoration of self-respect); enhancing mastery (including the accessing of social support); and facilitating the creation of meaning (in the context of existing belief systems). The model has been documented[45] and appears to work well based on practitioner and client reports, but has not been subject to any control-based or comparative research. It has been informally adopted by several non-government organisations (NGOs) and welfare bodies and is one of the main forms of counselling offered at the Trauma Clinic of the CSVR in Johannesburg, one of the few trauma-focused service organisations in the country.

There are other authors who have written about the benefits of an integrated approach to trauma work and have identified 'common ingredients' that appear to make trauma interventions successful. In a well-observed paper, Prout and Schwarz,[46] having reviewed the range of trauma intervention approaches available at the time, suggest that trauma interventions generally embrace the following principles: supporting adaptive coping skills; normalising trauma-related symptoms and feelings; decreasing avoidance of traumatic reminders; altering maladaptive attributions of meaning; and facilitating integration of the self (bringing together all the memories, feelings and thoughts about the trauma that the person may have split off from consciousness in order to defend themselves from the anxiety associated with these). Raphael and Wilson similarly comment that the benefits of trauma treatment pertain to 'helping the individual to confront what has happened; expression of feeling associated with the event; construction of meaning; and gaining practical and cognitive mastery'.[47] It seems then that there is considerable agreement about what 'ingredients' make good trauma treatment and that therapists might be well informed by holding these over-arching guidelines in mind in making decisions about how best to assist clients.

The neoterics or power therapies
Although not widely used in South Africa and lacking empirical or practical validation in many instances, the power therapies are worth mentioning, as these methods of intervention are employed by some practitioners in the country and are seen to promise fast alleviation of symptoms. In surveying some several hundred practitioners in the United States about trauma treatment approaches that they found had assisted with quick symptom reduction in a short number of sessions, Figley and Carbonell[48] identified four such approaches. These were Eye Movement Desensitisation and Reprocessing (EMDR), Traumatic Incident Reduction (TIR), Visual Kinaesthetic Dissociation (VKD) and Thought Field Therapy (TFT). All four approaches involve pairing of revisited trauma imagery under structured conditions with some anxiety-counteracting input, and so could perhaps be broadly viewed as 'exposure techniques', involving desensitisation to traumatic material. VKD has its origins in Neurolinguistic Programming (NLP) and TFT in applied kinesiology, but as exposure-based approaches

they could be viewed as broadly behaviour therapy-oriented. They are technique-based approaches, which is perhaps both their strength and limitation. The therapist takes a very active role in directing the process and the treatment is standard for every client, which is what is sometimes discomforting for both clients and therapists. In practice those trained in such techniques in South Africa tend to use them as part of a broad repertoire of available approaches, preferring to work in a more relational and case-based way with trauma clients. In focusing on symptom reduction there is little attention to meaning-making or integration of the trauma into life experience. EMDR is the most widely used and best researched of the power therapies and so will be discussed in more detail. In fact, some clinicians might contest its inclusion under the category of 'neoteric', viewing EMDR as a mainstream CBT approach or method within its own right.

EMDR[49] is a technique-based therapy approach that has become very popular in the United Kingdom and United States, and has proponents in South Africa since international practitioners come out regularly to offer training in the method to professionals at fairly substantial cost. The method was developed by Francine Shapiro almost by chance after a link was made between the stimulation of saccadic or rapid eye movements and the reduction of anxiety. EMDR has been categorised as a CBT intervention, since it involves elements of desensitisation and cognitive restructuring, but tends to be viewed as a distinct treatment based on neurological processing that is not yet fully understood. Because there has been considerable controversy about the method, it has been well researched and results have generally been positive in terms of beneficial outcomes. However, it is not conclusively established as to what actually produces therapeutic change and the necessity of rapid eye movement as part of the process has even been questioned.[50] There is a fairly lengthy assessment process that takes place before treatment is initiated and in many instances considerable insight occurs in this assessment phase. It is suggested that part of the success of EMDR might lie in its efficacy as a distraction technique, requiring the person to simultaneously focus on traumatic material and the task at hand (visually tracking the hand movement of the therapist). Despite considerable debate about what makes it work and whether it deserves its positive reputation, EMDR continues to be widely used and is the treatment of choice for many practitioners overseas. In South Africa many therapists are sceptical of the approach and, as with the other power therapies, are concerned about its overly technical base and its indiscriminate application. However, there are also proponents of EMDR, although it is perhaps not as widely practiced as it might be were the training not so expensive and, therefore, fairly elitist. Since the second phase of EMDR training is focused on working with more serious posttraumatic pathology (such as Dissociative Disorders), the training is also restricted to people with professional clinical training in psychology and medicine.

Having covered short term trauma intervention approaches in some depth the next section deals with longer term approaches.

Long-term approaches

Long term approaches to trauma therapy, that is, therapy of several months or years duration, tends to be oriented to more complex cases of trauma, for example early childhood trauma, and to more intractable cases of PTSD. Two main approaches are referred to here, psychodynamic or psychoanalytic trauma treatment and multi-dimensional treatment. Although CBT treatment can clearly be extended into longer-term intervention, it is generally intended as a short to medium term time-limited intervention. Psychodynamic approaches, on the other hand, are conventionally long-term oriented with an expectation that clients (or patients, as they are often referred to) will be in psychotherapy or analysis for years.

Psychodynamic treatment

As alluded to previously, the early history of psychoanalysis is strongly associated with the exploration of psychological trauma. Subsequently, however, the analytic movement's emphasis on unconscious, intra-psychic functioning and on the role of transference and counter-transference in effecting psychotherapeutic change, has meant that traumatic stress cases have sometimes been viewed as unsuitable for psychodynamic therapy. Nevertheless, there is a trauma service associated with the Tavistock Clinic in London, one of the most established psychodynamic psychotherapy training centres in the world. Caroline Garland, a key practitioner within this service, has edited a book which provides a basis for understanding psychodynamic approaches to trauma work, titled *Understanding trauma: a psychoanalytical approach*.[51]

Although there are different perspectives on mechanisms of traumatisation and related treatment within the psychodynamic community, some common elements will be outlined. Within this framework the subjective interpretation of the event by the patient is strongly emphasised, based on the assumption that the trauma experience will be shaped by, and mapped onto, prior life experiences, particularly fearful or disturbing experiences. Thus each individual's experience of a traumatic event is understood to be unique and the meaning of the incident can only be fully appreciated by exploring both conscious and unconscious associations to the trauma. In addition, the way in which the traumatic experience is processed will be shaped by the person's previous defensive style and intra-psychic dynamics. For example, a person who has a very harsh superego or internally judgmental aspect to their personality may struggle much more with surviving an incident in which a colleague was killed than someone with a more benign superego. It is also assumed that the manner in which the person deals with the trauma afterwards will reflect the health of their internal 'objects', which in part represent the kinds of blueprints for dealing with anxiety and danger that have been laid down by early experiences with significant caretakers.

Further, it is assumed that the trauma survivor's relationship with the therapist will also reflect these kinds of early 'object' relationships. For example, a client who has had the experience of a very fragile mother, who seemed overwhelmed by any demands made by her child, might choose to hide some of the worst aspects of the trauma incident in therapy, assuming that he or she can only be helped if they bring what is manageable to the therapist (who is unconsciously associated with the vulnerable mother). Drawing on a related idea, Herman reminds therapists that they should not always assume that traumatised clients share the perception of therapy as a benign process and suggests that for those who have been previously abused the therapist can sometimes be experienced as helpful, but can also be experienced as an abuser, a seducer or an impotent bystander.[52] Feelings from the past may be transferred onto the therapist in the present, and in the case of trauma, the strength of violations that the patient has experienced may sometimes mean that aspects of the trauma situation are unconsciously replayed in therapy.[53]

As should be evident from this brief discussion of psychoanalytic perspectives on trauma, the working through of material in therapy at this level can take considerable time. The early phase of therapy involves forming a good working relationship so that when the more in depth trauma-focused work needs to be done the therapeutic bond or alliance is strong enough to sustain the patient through the difficult process. It is also suggested that the therapist needs to play a strongly 'containing' role in therapy,[54] with the word 'containment' understood in a specific sense. It is the therapist's role (in parallel to that of a mother with a distressed infant) to be able to tolerate the most difficult and unmanageable feelings and sensations associated with the trauma, to be able to reflect upon and make sense of these, and then to be able to help the patient to symbolise this material and put it into words. This is perhaps a different way of understanding the benefit that the client may feel in talking through or narrating the trauma experience in depth to the therapist. It has also been proposed by psychodynamic therapists influenced by a 'Self Psychology' orientation that early work in trauma therapy with patients who have been severely abused and are not very stable, should consist of ego strengthening or assistance in developing 'self capacities'.[55] For example, a client may need to learn how to tolerate being alone, or to ask for help when fearful, before any processing of anxiety-provoking trauma memories can be introduced. While this might be seen as similar to teaching a client anxiety management techniques in CBT, self capacities are seen as deeper aspects of personality rather than as techniques that can be employed after some training. Again, it is apparent that working with complex trauma cases in this way might take years rather than weeks.

There is little research that systematically documents the impact of long-term psychodynamic therapy for trauma compared with other interventions, perhaps because of the highly individualised nature of the work with each case. However, there are some very compelling case studies documented in the psychoanalytic literature (for example in

Garland's book, referred to earlier). Much of the work in long-term psychodynamic treatment of trauma is about meaning-making and draws upon some of the understandings outlined in Chapter 4.

Multi-dimensional treatment

A second form of long-term therapy for trauma could perhaps best be termed multi-dimensional, since in some instances of treatment of more complex or intractable forms of trauma several different approaches and interventions might be used in combination. An individual may, for example, be involved in individual therapy, couple counselling (to deal with the relational impact of their trauma symptoms) and group therapy (to gain social support for their difficulties). Services for war veterans in the United States span these kinds of treatment inputs. In many instances trauma treatment with more marginalised populations extends beyond conventional forms of psychotherapy into psychosocial support, such as support in job-seeking.

Treatment for refugee victims of torture in specialist centres in Europe and England involves input from a multi-disciplinary team, including psychiatrists, psychologists, physiotherapists, social workers and others. For example, the Medical Foundation in the United Kingdom[56] and the treatment centres associated with the International Rehabilitation Council for Torture Victims (IRCT)[57] offer such multi-faceted intervention. Treatment may involve medication as well as physical and psychological rehabilitation. A central aspect of treatment for such populations is often some sort of occupational deployment or skills training, as it is recognised that trauma recovery is in part dependent upon the restitution of a sense of self-reliance and self-sufficiency. Long-term psychotherapy is but one aspect of a multi-dimensional intervention and the focus of the therapy may change over time to assist the client not only to process the past trauma but also to deal with its indirect effects in the present, including adjustment to very changed life circumstances. South Africa is one of five sites at present involved in piloting a torture treatment programme based on IRCT protocols.

While treatment facilities for African refugees in South Africa tend to be much more modest than those just described, there are attempts to work in a multi-dimensional way with psychiatrists, social workers, psychologists and lawyers often collaboratively assisting asylum seekers and refugees. Therapy with such refugees is often of extended duration as therapists attempt to support clients to establish some sort of daily stability and meaningful existence, whilst at the same time assisting them to process the experiences that led them to flee their country of origin and to manage more classic trauma symptoms.[58]

A further example of the employment of such a multi-dimensional therapy approach was a psychosocial programme aimed at ex-combatants run jointly by Technikon South Africa and the CSVR. Over about a six-month period, ex-combatants from the former liberation movements, who were unemployed at the time, received skills training in a number of trades and simultaneously attended a structured group-therapy programme aimed at trauma resolution, psychoeducation, exploration of identity, self-insight and social skills development. Several participants also chose to engage in additional individual therapy to explore issues that had come up in the groups in greater depth. Although the job placement aspect of the programme was not as successful as hoped, the evaluations of the psychosocial intervention was generally very positive.[59] It is sometimes important for skills development to supplement trauma work in order for people in deprived communities to attach value to psychotherapy. Complementing this perspective is the idea that highly traumatised and symptomatic individuals need psychotherapy if they are to be optimally able to make use of training, service and work opportunities.

It is evident that multi-dimensional long-term therapy for PTSD and traumatic stress can take both more conventional forms, in the employment of multiple and complementary psychotherapeutic interventions, or less traditional, more socially oriented forms, in the sense of addressing social and community needs as part and parcel of trauma intervention. In the case of the latter types of intervention there is a strong overlap or synthesis between psychotherapeutic and community psychology modes of intervention. However, further discussion of community-level interventions that do not necessarily entail traditional psychotherapy is warranted in a subsequent section.

Pharmacotherapy

Having looked extensively at primarily individual psychotherapeutic approaches to dealing with traumatic stress it is important to acknowledge that although psychotherapy is generally recognised as the treatment of choice for traumatic stress,[60] there is also evidence that pharmacotherapy, usually employed in conjunction with psychotherapy, can be of benefit to those suffering from PTSD and related conditions. Psychiatric medication is sometimes employed explicitly to assist the process of psychotherapy, particularly exposure-oriented therapy, helping the patient to manage the re-experiencing symptoms and the associated anxiety that often increase initially in such treatments.[61] 'For example, antidepressants can dampen down involuntary re-experiencing symptoms such as flashbacks and nightmares, particularly when used in conjunction with insight oriented therapy. By modifying involuntary re-experiencing symptoms that follow intense and painful memories in psychotherapy, antidepressants allow patients to more freely experience, work through and master the trauma.'[62] Psychotherapy and pharmacotherapy can thus be used in complementary ways in the treatment of PTSD

As advances in brain imaging technology allow the neurobiology of traumatic stress to be increasingly better understood, the use of medication in treating specific aspects of PTSD is becoming refined. However, there are some general trends which are briefly summarised here. 'With very few exceptions (e.g., sleep disturbances, bipolar disorder), the experts prefer the selective serotonin reuptake inhibitors (SSRIs) as the first line of treatment.'[63] Thus PTSD is generally treated with similar medication to that used to treat depressive disorders and this tends to be the first kind of medication prescribed for people suffering from PTSD (despite its categorisation as an anxiety disorder in diagnostic systems). In cases of ASD it is not uncommon for general practitioners (GPs) to prescribe tranquillisers (or anxiolytic medications) and sleeping tablets or sedatives. While these medications may assist with the immediate or short-term control of symptoms, they need to be carefully managed so as not to create dependence and also so as not to suppress the processing of traumatic material required for longer-term adjustment. Suppression of traumatic symptoms or memories is not desirable, medical support should rather be designed to assist with optimal processing of trauma experiences. It should also be recognised that the conditions that are commonly comorbid with PTSD, such as depression or substance dependence, may also require pharmacologic treatment.

A somewhat more differentiated discussion of drug treatments for PTSD suggests the following in terms of symptom management. 'Medications most often prescribed include antidepressant, andrenergic blockers, benzodiazepines and anticonvulsants ... Among antidepressants, serotonergic antidepressants have demonstrated efficacy in treating core PTSD symptoms when prescribed at higher doses for 5-8 weeks ... Tricyclic antidepressants have alleviated intrusive symptoms, sleep disturbances, anxiety and depression, but have not reliably reduced avoidance.'[64] In further summarising the results of several clinical trials, Tucker and Trautman also indicate that adrenergic blockers may be used to treat strong arousal symptoms, lithium or mood stabilisers to treat impulsivity and labile mood, anticonvulsants to reduce constant hyperarousal, and benzodiazepines to treat severe anxiety and panic attacks.

It is apparent that medication is part of the repertoire of interventions available to treat ASD and PTSD and that the prescription of drugs in such cases is becoming increasingly refined. It seems most useful for medical and psychological practitioners to work collaboratively in planning optimal treatment for clients. Writing from a psychotherapeutic point of view, Southwick and Yehuda[65] provide an interesting critical reflection about how the prescription of medication may play a role in the therapeutic relationship and what meaning clients may attach to this. They stress that therapists need to be both open to the use of medication and mindful of the impact of the introduction of medication into an existing therapeutic partnership or treatment regime.

In South Africa it seems that the majority of trauma cases, particularly ASD cases, are treated by psychotherapists or counsellors, including professionals and volunteers. It is primarily in cases of chronic or severe PTSD that psychiatric intervention is introduced (or takes primacy) or in cases where serious comorbid psychiatric conditions are present. Few pure PTSD cases are treated as in-patients and in most cases medication is managed on an out-patient basis. Psychotherapists tend to refer clients for psychiatric assessment when symptoms appear intractable and particularly when anxiety or depressive symptoms become debilitating. In rare instances, clients being treated for PTSD may manifest psychotic symptoms and require hospitalisation. For example, a Rwandan refugee woman who had witnessed the killing of family members and had been raped in a refugee camp prior to coming to South Africa, began to describe 'hearing voices' and to demonstrate bizarre behaviour, following an assault in this country, and required psychiatric referral and hospitalisation. Given the large numbers of people affected by traumatic incidents in the country, it is the minority who see psychiatrists, and it is not uncommon for GPs and traditional healers to be the practitioners who prescribe medical and physical treatments. In general, there is reasonable collaboration between medical and psychosocial practitioners with cross-referral taking place, although there is still some ignorance concerning the fact that both psychotherapy and pharmacotherapy can be of benefit and that treatment for traumatic stress generally requires some form of counselling or psychotherapy.

Group Psychotherapy

There are three main forms of widely used group psychotherapy for trauma: psychodynamic, cognitive behavioural and supportive.[66] Groups are usually offered to people suffering from the same kind of trauma, for example, rape, combat stress or a terminal illness diagnosis. One of the difficulties in forming such groups is that individuals may be at very different stages in the processing of their experiences, but group treatment is economical and has particular merits. The main benefits of group psychotherapy lie in the support that such groups can offer (beyond that of the therapist and existing networks) and the degree to which they aid in the reduction of stigma by facilitating the sharing of common experiences and reactions. Normalisation of trauma reactions is very powerful in group therapy, since members find that they can identify with others' accounts. In some cases relational networks are created that are sustained outside of therapy. In a group conducted for asylum seekers traumatised by the 9/11 attacks in New York City. participants reported that the building of social bonds with others in a similar predicament was one of the most beneficial aspects of group attendance.[67]

While each of the three approaches differs in focus, 'the ultimate goal for both psychodynamic and cognitive behavioural group therapy is for group members to gain "authority" over traumatic material so that it no longer becomes a dominant factor in their lives'. [68] In contrast, supportive group therapy is generally present-centred and aimed at management of everyday issues as well as social and interpersonal skills development. Research has indicated that all three forms of group psychotherapy are associated with improvements, with CBT approaches again demonstrating the most conclusive benefits.[69]

Alongside these more conventional forms of group psychotherapy there are a range of other approaches, some of which appear to wax and wane in terms of popularity. One alternative form of group psychotherapy that has been offered for several years in South Africa, initially under the auspices of the National Peace Accord Trust (NPAT), is what is known as 'Wilderness Therapy'.[70] Originally developed by two psychologists in conjunction with an ex-member of one of the township paramilitary structures, Wilderness Therapy for traumatised groups adapted the principles of eco-psychological, Jungian-oriented, wilderness therapy to meet the needs of local groups. Selected groups of trauma survivors are taken into natural areas, such as the Cedarberg or the Drakensberg, to take part in a ritualised process of self and group discovery over several days. Amongst other benefits there was the development of self-reliance and mastery through negotiation of physically and emotionally challenging tasks; the development of trust through sharing and team-building processes; and the development of self-reflection, introspection and meaning-making in the face of time spent in isolation and against a vast natural backdrop. The physicality of the therapy is seen as important in that trauma experiences are understood as being 'locked in the body' as well as the mind. 'The physical obstacles, challenges, failures and achievements are understood as impacting directly on, and involving completely, their psychological equivalents.'[71] The programme also draws on notions of the collective unconscious and Jungian archetypes and brings all these aspects to bear in the facilitation of trauma processing. Initially it was primarily men who had taken part in military and paramilitary structures during the anti-apartheid struggle (sometimes from opposing political structures) who took part in the trails. Subsequently the programme was broadened to cater for adolescents at risk, sex workers and other marginalised populations, losing some of its narrower traumatic stress focus.[72] Anecdotal reports indicate that there is considerable benefit for both individuals and communities ensuing from such programmes. In some respects this more ritualised form of healing parallels reports of the use of American Indian Sweat Lodge practices in the treatment of Vietnam War veterans. It is argued that traditional practices geared towards taking community members through rites of passage can be adapted to take traumatised groups through some sort of trauma cleansing, healing and transcendence process.

Other alternative forms of group psychotherapy draw on creative and active participation models. For example, there is a form of psychodrama specifically oriented to trauma work offered by the Spiral Therapy group that involves using trained team support in the group enactment of trauma. Some Spiral Therapy trainers visited South Africa a few years ago to demonstrate and train NGO members in the method, but the approach does not seem to have taken off widely, despite the fact that enactment of trauma seems to be a natural form of facilitating catharsis and working through. There are also trauma healing groups involving collective creative activities, such as the production of art work or the workshopping of short plays for performance. South African counsellors and community members have shown considerable innovation in this regard, in part out of necessity and in part out of recognition of the richness of local cultural resources. Many of these innovative approaches are not widely documented and one of the tasks of the National Network of Trauma Service Providers set up in the late 1990s, known as *Themba Lesizwe*,[73] was to gather and document the range of treatment approaches being used in the country and to establish guidelines for best practice. Unfortunately the network has been terminated due to lack of funding but the capacity for creative intervention development continues. This is seen, for example, in the range of group psychotherapeutic interventions that have been developed to work with issues associated with HIV and AIDS.

In addition to the formally constituted groups (both conventional and alternative) facilitated usually by at least one or two professional therapists, there are forms of trauma therapy that make use of peer support and networks. One such organisation in South Africa is 'Compassionate Friends', a group set up to support people suffering from bereavement related to the loss of a child, usually under traumatic circumstances. The network is made up of similarly bereaved people who hold group meetings and also offer one-on-one support. The organisation's underlying philosophy is that people with similar experiences who have had time to work through their trauma and bereavement may be well placed to assist those who are newly traumatised. There is a similar support network for women recently diagnosed with breast cancer, also staffed by breast cancer survivors. Self-help or peer support groups have also been established by ex-combatants in South Africa and by survivors of human rights violations in the form of the organisation known as *Khulumani*.[74] Friedman[75] observes that because of its non-professional roots, peer counselling has not been well researched, but comments that ongoing involvement in such structures and initiatives suggests that those that flourish must have benefit for participants. Given the constraints to offering professional assistance to the South African population as a whole, self-help initiatives for trauma survivors are a welcome addition to overstretched state and NGO services, provided they are ethically managed. Many of these peer support groups make use of professional input on an ad-hoc basis or are supported free of charge by professionals as a social service to the community.

Common Mechanisms and Best Practice

The discussion of individual and group therapy for traumatic stress has covered considerable ground. At this point it might be helpful to offer a short discussion on what aspects of psychotherapy have generally been found to be beneficial or form part of what has become known as 'evidence-based practice' or 'best practice'.

There is generally consensus amongst trauma treatment service providers that the establishment of a strong, trustworthy therapeutic relationship is crucial to the success of therapy. In addition:

Regardless of the type of psychotherapy used, certain elements of psychotherapy are especially important in engaging and maintaining patients in treatment of PTSD, such as establishing a strong therapeutic rapport, confronting denial, setting limits for behaviours such as substance abuse and self-injurious acts, and emphasizing the 'here and now' as well as processing the trauma.[76]

This quotation summarises some of the important elements in creating what could be termed the 'frame' or context within which effective psychotherapy can take place. Assuming the establishment of a good, containing, hope-instilling therapeutic relationship, research into different modalities has established that some aspects of therapy appear to be particularly beneficial in terms of specific symptoms. 'Overall the most highly recommended psychotherapy techniques are anxiety management, cognitive therapy, exposure therapy and psychoeducation. Play therapy is recommended for children. The experts reported three preferences for treating specific PTSD symptoms: Exposure therapy for intrusive thoughts, flashbacks, trauma-related fears, and avoidance; cognitive therapy for guilt and shame symptoms; and anxiety management for hyperarousal and sleep disturbances.'[77] Psychoeducation is an important supplementary therapeutic mechanism but is generally not viewed as a sufficient treatment in and of itself.[78]

In general it is also well established that psychotherapy is beneficial in the treatment of psychological trauma and PTSD. 'A meta-analysis of controlled clinical trials of psychotherapeutic treatment for PTSD, including cognitive behavioural and psychodynamic modalities, in both group and individual settings, demonstrated significant reduction of symptoms with no decay in effects on follow-up (Sherman, 1998).'[79] Tucker and Trautman[80] also go on to summarise the findings of a study conducted into the progress of 459 people with PTSD, indicating that psychotherapeutic treatment significantly reduced the duration of PTSD in this group. It is generally widely accepted then that traumatic stress conditions are amenable to psychotherapy and that a range of interventions offer established benefit. This having been said, it is important to raise some further contextually relevant issues that influence the practice and provision of trauma treatment in South Africa. These considerations reflect both caveats to accepted wisdoms about trauma intervention and special contributions that South African practitioners have made to the trauma field, spurred on by fairly unique contextual demands.

Treatment of Multiple and Continuous Traumatic Stress

An element that characterises much trauma work in South Africa is the fact that large numbers of clients suffer multiple traumatisation, being subject to a range of different traumatic events in their lives.[81] Alongside this is the fact that the recovery environment is often perceived as still dangerous and in reality may well be so. At the outset of the chapter it was emphasised that the creation of safety is almost a precondition for the introduction of trauma-focused psychotherapy. The provision of containment and stabilisation as essential for therapeutic benefit was reiterated in a number of subsequent sections, for example in relation to debriefing and self-psychology models of intervention. In South Africa, the establishment of this kind of safe, holding environment is sometimes not feasible, since, as noted in Chapter 3, many South Africans live in situations of continuous trauma exposure. Thus, many trauma survivors who present for treatment face the real prospect of future victimisation and cannot easily escape dangerous living circumstances. This is in part because of generally very high levels of violence in particular communities, but also because of inefficiencies, corruption, lack of capacity and lack of resources in the criminal justice system. To describe a case in point, a woman in her early twenties who had reported her rape by a taxi driver to the local police station found that initially her case report went missing. After making a second report her family home was visited by three associates of the taxi driver who threatened to assault family members if she did not withdraw the case. At the time of coming for counselling she had relocated to live with a friend in town but was afraid of being followed from her place of work and particularly concerned about the safety of her grandmother who reported a man loitering across the street from the family home. Such reports are not uncommon. During ongoing taxi route and drug dealing territory disputes there may be several assaults and murders, attacks on property and on family members, with those indirectly and directly involved feeling little sense of safety. Asylum seekers from other African countries are particularly vulnerable to continuous traumatic stress, with the prospect of xenophobic attacks, muggings and police raids on places of accommodation. One refugee client has reported three rapes or sexual assaults since coming to South Africa, in part, because of living a precarious existence on the streets of a major city. It is also not infrequent for clients to bring new traumatic experiences that have taken place during the course of psychotherapy to counselling, in one case a mugging that had just taken place on the way to therapy. Such accounts and client circumstances can be rather overwhelming for counsellors who may question whether there is any benefit in offering services in such circumstances, given the cardinal issue of safety in treatment. However, such clients also often desperately need support and look to counselling to help sustain them through such difficult experiences. See Box 5.1 for the findings of a recent study[82] into observations concerning the counselling of refugee clients in South Africa, many of whom could be viewed as continuous traumatic stress cases.

Straker and the Sanctuaries Counselling Team,[83] who developed the concept of 'continuous traumatic stress' in the context of their work with political activists, recognised that they had an important role to play for the traumatised activists who sought out their assistance, but also realised that their therapeutic input needed to be tailored to take account of their particular circumstances. Many of the principles informing their intervention still have bearing for working generally with clients in non-containing or risky environments. Although it is not possible to do justice to the full content of Straker et al.'s[84] article on continuous traumatic stress, some important features are highlighted. Recognising that clients in this kind of circumstance might not be predictable in their attendance of therapy it is proposed that every session be treated as a potentially stand-alone intervention. Trust may need to be rebuilt at each new appointment and sessions should be terminated or 'closed' with particular care, ensuring as far as possible that the client feels adequately contained and able to operate in the

Box 5.1

Therapeutic issues in working with African 'refugee' clients in South Africa

Grootenhuis (2006) conducted a qualitative research study[83] into counselling services for refugees by interviewing four refugee clients and four therapists who had worked with refugees at the CSVR about their experiences. The focus was on what had been found to be beneficial, where difficulties had been encountered and what particular dilemmas psychotherapists faced in such work. The following dilemmas were commonly reported by the therapists:

Therapist dilemmas

(1) Therapists had difficulty in straddling supportive and exploratory therapeutic objectives and interventions given the unstable living conditions of asylum seeking clients.

(2) Therapists found existing trauma therapy models either inadequate or overly rigid for work with such clients.

(3) In diagnosing clients, therapists experienced difficulty in distinguishing between personality and situational dimensions, particularly with respect to anxious, depressed and paranoid presentations.

(4) Therapists experienced role conflict with respect to potentially contaminating the therapeutic alliance in feeling compelled to offer clients practical and social support.

(5) Role conflict contributed to a lack of team cohesion and feelings of inadequacy.

(6) The powerfully dependent transference of refugees was experienced as burdensome.

(7) The truthfulness of clients' accounts was sometimes in question given refugee perceptions of therapists' capacity to influence decisions about their status and potential resettlement, creating some difficulties in terms of relational congruence.

(8) Therapists had strong counter-transference feelings about the victimisation and lack of institutional support faced by refugees in South Africa, including feelings of guilt, anger, frustration, despondency, anxiety and shame by association.

(9) Therapists found such work physically tiring.

(10) Therapists found reward in being of some assistance and in witnessing the resilience of refugee clients.

context they return to. The therapist may also allow for the extension of the time of sessions beyond the conventional hour.[85]

Straker et al. argue that therapists need to recognise that, in general, the client's defences should not be tampered with as they are necessary for ongoing survival. At the same time it may well still be important to assist the client to process traumatic experiences by talking about them. This discussion of events should as far as possible be restricted to factual and cognitive aspects, consciously steering away from emotional, sensory and physical associations. A strong focus of the therapy should be on coping resources and the mechanisms that clients can employ to manage their fears and the real threats in their environment. The therapist may help the client to distinguish as far as possible between real and imagined threat, as opposed to potential risk (in other words, the enhancement of discriminating capacities). Realistic fear and distress is not minimised and survival strategies are explicitly explored. The therapist attempts to hold realistic hope for the client. At the CSVR, therapists talk about helping the client to find 'islands of safety', representing mental spaces that feel uncontaminated by daily stressors. Such mental spaces may be achieved through training in relaxation techniques, guided fantasy, prayer or taking part in particular activities (such as playing sport or attending a religious ceremony). In CBT terms, it could be argued that much greater weight is placed on anxiety management, as opposed to exposure techniques, with cognitive restructuring work oriented towards realistic appraisal and acknowledgement of what internal and external resources are available for coping with potential threats. Such psychotherapy might also be subsumed under the label of 'supportive psychotherapy'. However working with continuous traumatic stress may call for some engagement with traumatic material as discussed above, as opposed to restricting work to everyday issues. The aim of such interventions may well be modest, such as the emotional 'holding' of the person in the situation and the prevention of the development of serious pathology, such as major depression, dissociative conditions or psychotic breakdown.

In addition to their therapeutic role, therapists may find themselves taking on advocacy roles, becoming involved in assisting clients to relocate or to better access the criminal justice system and other formal systems of protection. This has implications for the therapeutic relationship and therapist capacity that need to be carefully thought through, but the adoption of advocacy roles may feel more congruent for therapists in such contexts.[86] With such explicit understandings in mind, therapists may be able to continue to intervene without feeling completely de-skilled or helpless. While such demands have been strongly characteristic of much trauma intervention in South Africa, it is apparent that most contexts of civil conflict, war, political repression and endemic community violence, throw up similar challenges and have produced similar observations about how to promote resilience in such circumstances.

Traditional / Indigenous Practices

A further interesting and somewhat unique aspect of trauma intervention in South Africa is the fact that traditional African healers play a significant role as traumatic stress practitioners. We have seen in Chapter 4 that individuals seek to make meaning of traumatic events and that such meaning is often socially and culturally located. For example, we noted that in traditional African belief systems misfortune is generally viewed as caused by some agent or set of events, rather than as purely accidental. At the risk of over-generalisation, traumatic events are often understood to stem from either human or ancestral agency, particularly when multiple misfortunes have occurred, and two common explanations offered for misfortune are bewitchment and displeasure on the part of ancestors.[87] If such cultural attributions for traumatic events are dominant for an individual, they are likely to seek the assistance of a traditional practitioner who may help identify the source of the troubles and prescribe certain medicines, practices or rituals to overcome the adversity. For example, in the case that misfortune is attributed to disrespect of ancestors it is very common for clients to be instructed to perform some kind of ritual slaughter of an animal. It is often suggested that the trauma will remain unresolved and further misfortune follow, in the absence of such rituals. Given the powerful impact of trauma, it is not unusual for westernised African people to entertain more traditional beliefs when they attempt to make sense of such events. It is therefore important that therapists take account of such belief systems and are open to the fact that many African people not only consult traditional practitioners as their healer of choice, but also that some clients may use 'westernised' and traditional services concurrently. In many instances such treatment is complementary but psychotherapists may sometimes be called upon to negotiate tensions between different explanatory frameworks.[88] It is also worth reiterating that traditional healers represent a significant group of trauma interventionists in South Africa, albeit that their treatment appears to differ quite strongly from western therapeutic approaches and has not been subject to scientific validation.[89]

Social Alienation as a Product of Traumatisation

One of the other features that many trauma practitioners have observed in South Africa is that traumatised individuals often tend to become increasingly prejudiced, alienated and critical of government and society in general. Victims of crime, in particular, perceive a lack of capacity or even a lack of will on the part of the criminal justice system to protect them, to curb crime and to apprehend and punish offenders. This perception in turn appears to contribute to disillusionment, hopelessness and depression that extend beyond conventional trauma symptomology, as well as to retributive acts and vigilantism. In some instances, disinvestment leads to emigration or relocation. A very common response amongst trauma survivors is an increase in racism or inter-group prejudice.[90] Following counsellor observations about the difficulty of engaging with the extremity of racism and prejudice that commonly emerges in trauma counselling in South Africa, Benn[91] undertook research with victims of violent attacks who volunteered to be interviewed about self-observed alterations to their race or group-based attitudes, including the entertainment of xenophobia, anti-black and anti-ethnic sentiments. A number of these interviewees (both 'black' and 'white') volunteered that they had experienced extreme feelings of anxiety, fear, anger, hatred, suspicion and mistrust towards groups of people who they associated with their attackers, consequent on their traumatisation. They had also found themselves entertaining increasingly negative stereotypes about such groups of people, including ideas that they were inherently violent, cruel, inhumane, primitive, animal-like and dangerous. For victims who had previously held liberal or anti-racist positions such alterations to their schemas were very uncomfortable. These ideas and sentiments often surface in psychotherapy and present ethical, technical and counter-transferential dilemmas for psychotherapists.[92] Counsellors and therapists struggle to know how to engage with such content. Given the extremity of traumatisation and frequently regressed presentation of traumatised clients, it may feel uncontaining and counter-therapeutic to explore and challenge such material. Therapists are trained to respect client autonomy, including the respect of a client's value system and may see such intervention as a form of consciousness-raising exceeding their brief as psychotherapists. Nevertheless it is possible to understand such alterations to attitudes as a pathological response to trauma, either in terms of stimulus over-generalisation or more complicated unconscious defensive processes of splitting, projection and displacement, and therefore to understand it to be a therapeutic imperative to intervene to change such responses if possible. In two related studies investigating how non-professional trauma debriefers[93] and psychodynamically-oriented clinical psychologists[94] work with negative racial sentiments in traumatised clients in practice, both groups volunteered that they felt some personal discomfort not only in listening to such material but also in knowing how to separate out their own feeling or countertransference responses in order to appreciate how and when to intervene. Working with such prejudice and the disillusionment, social alienation and negativity described earlier, places considerable pressure on local psychotherapists. Such responses to trauma are clearly contextually informed and reflect responses to a transforming society in which social institutions and the nature of government have changed rapidly and dramatically over the past decade against a backdrop of a prior, shameful history of racial oppression. However, it could be argued that the world is rapidly transforming and there is clearly evidence of this kind of group prejudice occurring in response to violence in other parts of the world, such as the anti-Arab prejudice that has developed in response to the 9/11 attacks in America and the bombings in England in 2007. Contemporary trauma therapists are required to be reflective about their own values and sometimes to interrogate accepted wisdoms in responding to this 'politicised' element of trauma intervention. South Africa therapists may be well placed to lead the way in thinking through how to engage with such trauma responses.

Box 5.2

Negative racial sentiments amongst traumatised clients: observations and therapeutic implications

Case Example

In a study conducted by Benn in 2007, a woman who had been robbed and threatened, and whose husband had been shot and killed by a group of house breakers reported that her attitudes had altered in the following way:

I have always been very trusting and very comfortable, you know, I do not think that I would have behaved any different in a crowd situation with black people or white people. I would expect a white kid to pickpocket me just as readily as I would expect a black person to grab my handbag. I avoid them now, the idea of any physicality with them is like 'yuck', disgust ... and I do have a different perception of common everyday people I might encounter. I see the potential now for black men to be ruthless, callous and definitely not to live by the same human rules as I am and the abiding mass of people are. Okay. One change for me is that I now see the potential for damage and harm and danger in every black man I see.

Recognising the complexity of such a presentation in a context such as South Africa, it is nevertheless possible to see how the regression and traumatisation associated with violent attack or threat of attack leads to the employment of defences such as othering, distantiation, displacement, projection and splitting. There is clearly also evidence of over-generalisation and the surfacing of categoric and stereotypical ways of thinking. It is apparent that this victim of trauma remains imprisoned in a fearful world in which it is difficult to distinguish the good people from the bad people, and crude markers (such as skin colour) then become salient. Despite having received some trauma counselling it appears that her anxiety levels associated with the presence of black men are still very high and that the changes to her belief system or schemas are somewhat enduring. This poses questions as to how to work therapeutically with such material.

Therapists' Reflections

Therapists and counsellors indicated that they frequently encountered such kinds of sentiments in traumatised clients, often expressed with considerable intensity in early sessions in counselling. In Fletcher's 2007 study, it appears that therapists make informal assessments concerning, for example, how regressed the client is and whether they are still in the impact phase or have moved beyond this, whether the sentiments appear to be ego-syntonic or ego-dystonic in terms of client discomfort, whether there is an alteration to or a solidification of prior attitudes, whether the client has adequate support outside of therapy and how strong the therapeutic alliance is. This informs the decision as to whether it is appropriate to use a more challenging as opposed to a more reflective intervention (with concern in the latter case not to appear to legitimate prejudice).

I generally don't address racist material in therapy with a client who has been through a trauma. Often in the first week or two or three that will come with a lot of racism; a lot of anger is expressed in racism, the injustice of trauma is expressed in racism, but often that abates as part of the process of working through the trauma. I don't find that one necessarily has to address it directly. (Therapist 2)

When they decide to intervene in more challenging ways, therapists then generally chose one of two approaches. They may locate the prejudice at the level of a symptom and employ psychoeducation to reduce polarisation and over-generalisation.

On a level it is part of the desensitization process. Not everybody is a criminal. Not everybody of that race is worse than someone of another race. (Therapist 5)

Alternatively, psychodynamic therapists in particular might work more interpretively, linking such virulent content to underlying feelings of helplessness, rage and impotence.

If I am working with a client long term, it is all about the internal world, how do I relate? What their object relations are like, whether they have punitive objects because then often those prejudices are a way of making the self feel better in the world. Inevitably if you take them there, there is a very helpless, powerless, insecure child that you are dealing with. They were raised in a world where someone had to be the baddy. If I don't look like that then at least I have some good, at least I have some value. (Therapist 1)

Therapists recognised their own ambivalences in engaging with such material and the fact that, if left untreated, such elements of trauma impact may have not only personal but also societal consequences.

A person who is using primitive defences can actually be horrible to other people whether it is racist or whether it is just that they have got these bad objects and they hate them. If you look at a whole society doing that, the cost of it is huge, there is war. (Therapist 6)

It thus seems that careful attention to such material in therapy is important in the prevention of further spirals of violence, racism and prejudice and that therapists have moral as well as technical obligations and choices to make in this regard.

Community Interventions, Rituals And Memorials

A chapter covering traumatic stress treatment and intervention in South Africa would not be complete without some discussion of community-level interventions. While the subject of community interventions could comprise a chapter on its own, this sub-section provides some orientation to this level of input. Some aspects of community-level interventions have been discussed in the earlier section on group interventions, particularly the psychosocial aspects of such intervention. Wilderness therapy aimed at selected participants from communities in conflict could also be understood as a community intervention in some respects. However, it is important to recognise that some trauma interventions are targeted at large groups of people forming communities of various kinds, rather than at individually traumatised people within such groups. The indirect effects of traumatisation on the social networks of direct victims have been recognised, as has the fact that traumatic events often tear apart the social fabric of communities. Interventions are usually designed to collectively mark and mourn what has been lost and to recreate some sense of social cohesion.

Meintjes[95] describes such a community intervention project aimed at healing the trauma of communities affected by the extreme political violence that took place between African National Congress (ANC) and Inkatha Freedom Party (IFP) supporters in the period leading up to the first democratic elections in 1994. She documents the difficulties encountered in entering and gaining credibility in such communities in the face of very high levels of mistrust. She also describes the necessarily multi-faceted nature of such intervention, including occupational skills development, inter-group mediation, and psychoeducation, in addition to holding groups that were overtly therapeutic in orientation. It is apparent that a range of community practice skills is necessary for effective trauma intervention in such situations.

In addition to its other objectives, the South African TRC was intended partly as a trauma healing intervention at the level of communities and the nation as a whole. 'Despite its shortcomings, the process served as a public acknowledgement of the political and social nature of the context in which atrocities were committed and

119

individuals traumatised, and an impetus to create a new future in which racial conflicts would no longer result in tragic and needless conflict. The significance of the TRC as a social process towards healing has been widely acknowledged.'[96] At a social level, in keeping with aspects of individual trauma therapy, it was hoped that the surfacing of difficult, painful and horrific material would allow for collective catharsis and avoidance of suppression and repression of historical atrocities. This idea was complemented by an expectation of public and collective censure and apology as grounds for potential reconciliation. There have been numerous evaluations of aspects of the TRC with mixed findings about its ostensible strengths and weaknesses.[97] Nevertheless, as a model for reconciliation in previously conflict ridden societies, it has been drawn upon to inform similar processes in countries such as Northern Ireland, Rwanda and Sierra Leone. The TRC epitomises a societal level trauma intervention.

One of the outcomes of the TRC was restitution of both a material and symbolic nature. At a symbolic level, monuments have been erected to struggle heroes, and streets and geographical areas have been named after such individuals. Such initiatives represent further collective approaches to heal trauma through remembrance and homage. Such social symbols or markers have existed since time immemorial around the world, such as the tomb of the 'unknown soldier' and the many monuments and gardens of remembrance commemorating war victims. The declaration of 16 June as a public holiday in South Africa, recognising the tragic sacrifices made by Soweto school children in foregrounding the struggle against apartheid, is a further example of such social memorialisation. Public rituals on such days of remembrance serve to pay respect to those who suffered traumatisation and to emphasise the need to prevent future such tragedies through community solidarity and mindfulness of the implications of conflict. While trauma practitioners may not be directly involved in initiating healing at these kinds of meta-social levels, they may play a part in the discursive construction of such events and in optimising social healing.

It should be evident that there are many interlinking tiers of intervention for traumatised individuals, families, groups, communities and populations, and that individual healing often needs to be complemented by broader interventions and vice versa.

Conclusion

In concluding this chapter on trauma interventions, it is perhaps worth making mention of one more aspect and that is to note the impact of trauma work on practitioners. It is widely accepted that traumatic stress counselling is emotionally taxing for psychotherapists, evoking strong feelings and resulting sometimes in vicarious traumatisation, compassion fatigue and powerful countertransferences.[98] Volunteer counsellors may be at even more risk than professionals, given a lack of awareness of warning signs and potentially toxic effects. Self-care strategies, regular supervision, group support, time for debriefing and collective reflection are all useful in managing responses to such work. It has also been suggested that therapists might experience what could be called 'vicarious resilience' in doing trauma work as they bear witness to how traumatised people manage to survive and even transcend such life shattering experiences.

Despite some poverty in professional resources, South Africa has a strong trauma intervention history with evidence of considerable innovation and creativity. Given the importance of trauma treatment in trauma recovery, it is essential that services are maintained and expanded where possible. In agreement with Edwards,[99] it is also important that therapists research and document their practices so that ever more credible bases for intervention are consolidated.

Chapter 6

TRAUMA AND CHILDREN

Any book on traumatic stress in South Africa would be incomplete without attention to the traumatisation of children. Exposure to traumatic events is not restricted to adults who operate in the world outside of the family or home and it is common cause that children (ranging from infants to adolescents) are vulnerable to trauma stemming from exposure to a broad spectrum of events. Children in many instances are both direct and indirect victims of trauma and are frequently witnesses to violence enacted between adults in their environment. While children may have a range of coping capacities to deal with extreme stressors, the fact that aspects of their bodies, minds and brains are not fully developed means that they are often particularly vulnerable to the impact of trauma. In addition, they need to invest psychological resources in mastering normative developmental tasks and attempts to manage traumatic events may impede such development and lead to considerable strain. Many studies have shown that the impact of trauma at early stages of development can have a long-lasting impact on personality formation, behaviour and mental health. For example, it is now well established that adult abusers more frequently report having suffered abuse in their own childhoods than non-abusers.[1] A South

African-based study found that, along with several other conditions, exposure to traumatic life events and childhood PTSD were associated with the increased likelihood that the individual would not complete high school education.[2] Trauma in childhood may thus have both more immediate as well as long-term effects.

While children present with trauma responses that in many respects parallel those of adults, their response to traumatic incidents is strongly determined by their developmental stage and capacities. Thus anyone assessing or intervening with traumatised children needs to have a good understanding of normal developmental patterns.

Prevalence of Trauma and Posttraumatic Stress in Children

It is difficult to establish what percentage of children are exposed to traumatic events and just how many become disturbed as a consequence of this, given some of the problems in assessing exposure and levels of distress across situations and countries. Trauma exposure, for pre-school children, for example, is unlikely to come to the attention of outside authorities unless parents or caregivers report such exposure on behalf of the child. It is clear that the more violent and conflicted any society, the more children will be exposed to extraordinary life stressors. Given the history of strife in South Africa and the elevated crime and accident levels discussed in Chapter 2, it is to be anticipated that trauma exposure levels for South African children are high. Indeed, several studies of school-age children in South Africa have indicated that exposure to what might generally be considered *extraordinary* traumatising events, is actually normative in certain contexts. In a study comparing levels of exposure to traumatic events amongst South African and Kenyan youth, it was found that 80 per cent of these adolescents had been exposed to severe trauma at some point in their lives, either as direct victims or as witnesses.[3] A South African study conducted in Cape Town found that fifty-seven of the sixty children assessed (thirty school children from a violent area and thirty from a children's home in Khayelitsha) had witnessed violence and thirty-four had experienced violence themselves.[4] Another survey of 185 children at five township schools in Cape Town also found an extremely high rate of exposure to violence: 73 per cent of the children had witnessed someone being beaten up, 57 per cent had seen someone being attacked with a sharp weapon, 45 per cent had witnessed someone being threatened with a gun and 35 per cent had witnessed someone being killed in their neighbourhood.[5] Even in a survey of youth at private schools in Cape Town, trauma exposure levels were high, with 30 per cent reporting that they had been violently assaulted by a stranger and 48 per cent reporting an assault by someone known to them.[6] A further study conducted in a 'high-violence' area in Cape Town found that amongst the Grade 6 children assessed across five schools, well over half (68.44 per cent) reported exposure to violence either as victim and/or as witness.[7] And it is not only children in urban settings who are exposed to high levels of violence: a study of 148 children in a rural community in the Northern Province found that 67 per cent had experienced a traumatic event, either directly or as a witness.[8] These studies collectively suggest that by adolescence easily half the population of children in South Africa may have been exposed to a traumatic event either as a witness or direct victim. It is thus important to understand what the impact of such exposure might be and what scope there is for both preventive and secondary intervention.

While there are no groups of children who are necessarily exempt from trauma exposure, levels of exposure do appear to differ in relation to demographic features such as gender, race and class, and in relation to socio-political and historical circumstances. For example, 'minority' male youth in America seem to be exposed to more violent crime than their counterparts[9] and in the previously cited study comparing South African and Kenyan adolescents,[10] the Kenyan youth interestingly reported significantly higher levels of exposure to witnessing violence and physical and sexual assault, suggesting context-related differences in life circumstances. Some historical events clearly place large numbers of children at risk, such as wars, civil conflicts, genocides and mass displacement of people.[11] In countries at war, children become both direct victims of violence, as in the much publicised case of the child burn victim in Iraq, or indirect victims, in the sense of witnessing combat and conflict related atrocities. Children's lives are often further disrupted by family instability and the breakdown of health and educational structures. Children may also become orphaned, displaced or separated from families in the aftermath of major conflicts and there are large numbers of refugee children living in camps in many parts of Africa, some of these unaccompanied minors. Thus traumatic events may have effects beyond immediate shock and traumatisation, powerfully affecting the subsequent context within which a child continues to develop, and in this respect it is difficult to do justice to the full impact of traumatic events within the kinds of diagnostic systems available. For example, two little girls who had witnessed their abusive father beat and stab their mother to death were sent to live with relatives, having to then cope with traumatic bereavement, the incarceration of their father, and the adjustment of living in a new household with relatives who were traumatised themselves and felt over-burdened by the responsibility of taking care of them.

As discussed in Chapter 3, in relation to adult populations, children exposed to traumatic stressors may not always present with difficulties that can be categorised within the framework of ASD or PTSD. As will be discussed further later, children may show their distress in the form of physical symptoms, depression, anxiety, school problems and developmental difficulties, amongst others. When the impact of trauma is compounded by ongoing related difficulties, for example, the adjustment to living with relatives as in the case just mentioned, it may become difficult to separate out where the effects of a trauma begin and end for a particular child.

Bearing this difficulty of categorisation in mind it is still useful to look at some figures for those children who do meet diagnostic criteria for PTSD or other psychiatric disorders. Studies of different populations of traumatised children have found varying prevalence rates, some of these of considerable concern. In a fairly recent study looking at the impact of military violence on Palestinian children aged from six to sixteen years it was found that 54 per cent of the children appeared to be suffering from severe PTSD and 33.5 per cent from mild PTSD.[12] Thus, in this context of ongoing conflict, the majority of children were symptomatic. On the other hand, in examining the impact of a natural disaster, in the form of a hurricane, on a population of school-going children in America, the number of children meeting PTSD diagnostic criteria was just over 5 per cent.[13] A study conducted in Australia on children admitted to hospital after a traumatic injury found ASD in 10 per cent and PTSD in 13 per cent of these children[14] It is apparent that different stressors are more or less likely to cause significant levels of symptomatology amongst different groups of children. It seems that one factor may be the issue of whether events are accidental or deliberately inflicted and, as with adults, it appears that human-inflicted trauma may be more likely to produce disturbance in children and adolescents than traumas of natural or non-human origin.[15]

In South Africa, several studies have documented levels of distress in traumatised children. In the late 1980s and early 1990s, most of this research focused on assessing the consequences of political violence and civil unrest in the last years of apartheid. These studies relied largely on indirect means of assessing traumatic distress among children, such as parent or teacher observations of PTSD symptoms or the content of the drawings of very young children,[16] or else drew on in-depth interviews and case studies.[17] Findings from these studies indicated that a high percentage of younger children experienced various symptoms of posttraumatic stress, while older youth exposed to chronic political violence frequently presented with difficulties related to substance abuse and aggression.

Although political violence is no longer prevalent, we have seen in Chapter 2 and earlier in this chapter that many South African children continue to live in conditions of both domestic and community violence With the increasing availability of standardised measures for PTSD and other disorders in children in the past decade, more recent South African studies have been able to document the psychiatric impact of childhood trauma more precisely. In the 1997 study conducted in Khayelitsha, which utilised a structured PTSD questionnaire, a psychiatric diagnostic interview and a semi-structured clinical interview, it was established that 40 per cent of the sixty children assessed manifested symptoms consistent with some kind of DSM diagnosis and 21.7 per cent met the criteria for PTSD.[18] In the comparative study between Kenyan and South African adolescents referred to earlier, a standardised self-report measure of PTSD found that 22 per cent of the South African sample were at high risk for meeting the criteria for PTSD whereas only 5 per cent of the Kenyan pupils displayed symptoms consistent with the diagnosis, despite the fact that Kenyan adolescents reported higher levels of exposure to violence than their South African counterparts.[19] A study assessing psychopathology amongst a group of ninety-seven adolescents and children who attended a Youth Stress Clinic in South Africa found that 53 per cent reported sexual abuse and 63.8 per cent of these abused children presented with PTSD.[20] Some other studies of posttraumatic symptoms among school-age children in South Africa have yielded lower rates of risk for PTSD (such as 8 per cent in the study of children in the Northern Province[21] and 6 per cent of adolescents in the study of private schools in Cape Town[22]). In addition to PTSD, symptoms of depression, aggression and anxiety have also been found to be associated with exposure to trauma among South African children.[23] An important finding from a longitudinal study with over 600 South African children is that, for all children regardless of gender or income level, indirect exposure to violence (through witnessing and hearing about it) produces effects very similar to those that result from direct victimisation.[24]

Although the relationship between AIDS and traumatic stress is still under considerable debate, the loss of a parent or parents to AIDS is clearly a serious stressor that is affecting increasing numbers of South African children under the age of eighteen, with estimates of 1.15 million maternal orphans by the year 2015. Research into the psychological well-being of sixty Cape Town-based African children orphaned by AIDS indicated that '73 per cent scored above the cut-off for Post-traumatic Stress Disorder'.[25] This same study also cites research indicating that amongst a group of Congolese AIDS orphans the PTSD prevalence was 39 per cent.

It is apparent that exposure to traumatic events is a serious problem for South African children and youth and that some child populations in the country are at significant risk for the development of PTSD and other disturbances. While some of the worst effects of apartheid-era policies and practices on children (including overt forms of state repression and separation from migrant parents[26]) may no longer be affecting child populations, it is clear that there are other both new and old forms of trauma exposure that currently play a role in the lives of South African children. These include exposure to criminal and family violence, injury in motor vehicle accidents, high levels of sexual abuse and child rape, and the impact of AIDS.[27] All of these features of South African society, as discussed previously, create particular patterns of traumatisation and vulnerability.

Having established that children and adolescents are indeed amongst the victims of traumatic events in all societies, including in South Africa, and that varying and often high proportions of such children are at risk for the development of pathology, it is useful to perhaps make three further observations concerning prevalence and diagnosis. The first noteworthy observation is that across a range of research studies it appears that girl children, like their adult counterparts, appear to be generally more vulnerable to the development of traumatic stress symptoms and also that younger children may, similarly, be more at risk.[28] However, developmental issues will be discussed further later in the chapter. The second issue worth noting is that because of their limited verbal and reading ability it is difficult to assess the impact of traumatic events on very young children and researchers are generally obliged to rely on the observations and reports of caretakers in such cases. Generally trauma in children is assessed by means of interviews, self-report measures, caretaker reports and sometimes projective tests.[29] Some of the differences in findings as regards prevalence rates for PTSD across different populations are a consequence of using different measures and different cut-off points. School-going children are easier to access and study than younger children. Thirdly, it is worth emphasising that children can be exposed to both acute and chronic traumatic stressors and that, as with adults, these two 'types' of traumatisation may produce different outcomes. In addition to the kinds of traumatic incidents associated with sudden, unexpected or catastrophic events, children are also exposed to other more chronic destructive forces. These include most significantly physical and sexual abuse by parents, family members, family associates, teachers, care takers or acquaintances. Such abuse is often ongoing or involves multiple exposures, that is, the same traumatising experiences happen repetitively. This kind of chronic traumatic exposure is generally understood to evoke different kinds of responses and symptoms from once-off traumas. 'Among the symptoms found in children following traumas that are not included in the DSM-IV, PTSD diagnostic criteria are affect dysregulation, somatisation, loss of beliefs, dissociation, self-destructive behaviours, loss of faith in authority or adults, and unrelenting hopelessness.'[30] These kinds of symptom patterns are more common in child victims of prolonged traumas and parallel the kinds of conditions described as complex PTSD in adults, as discussed in Chapter 3 and further in the following section of this chapter.

From the discussion of prevalence of trauma exposure and symptomatology in a range of studies it is clear that children are vulnerable to PTSD, but this does not necessarily give a full picture as to how children who are traumatised might show their distress. The next section offers a more in-depth discussion of the presentation of traumatic stress in children.

The Impact of Different Forms of Trauma on Children

One of the trauma theorists who has researched and written about children over a considerable period of time is Lenore Terr. In an important paper she wrote in 1991 entitled *Childhood traumas: an outline and overview*,[31] she presents a sensitive and comprehensive discussion of the impact of trauma on children, based both on research and her extensive clinical practice. She offers a useful formulation in proposing that what she calls Type I and Type II Disorders need to be understood differently, the former representing responses to once-off or 'single blow' traumas and the latter a set of responses to multiple or long-standing traumas. Being bitten by a dog, for example, might evoke a Type I Disorder, but being sexually abused over several years would be more likely to result in a Type II Disorder.

The focus of this book is primarily on trauma as it would be experienced in Type I conditions, that is, on traumatisation in the face of unexpected, abnormal, catastrophic, life-threatening and injurious events. For this reason, the discussion of Type II Disorders is rather brief since it is difficult to do justice to the complicated factors involved in longer-term abuse or child exploitation situations. These kinds of traumas are likely to take place within some kind of system (such as the family) that then ideally needs to be understood and treated as a whole. Dealing with this kind of abuse may require structural interventions, such as the calling in of welfare, policing and legal services. However, in her discussion of Type II Disorders in children it is apparent that Terr[32] identifies responses that parallel those characteristic of adults with complex PTSD. Terr argues that for child victims of prolonged and repetitive trauma, in addition to dealing with the torment of every trauma experience, it is the *anticipation* of injury and traumatisation (the anticipatory anxiety) that has to be managed. This is often achieved through the use of numbing and detachment, the use of cutting-off defences that allow the child not to feel too intensely and to become almost immune to a pain they cannot escape. In order to survive in an environment in which they are often dependant on their abusers for material and psychological care, children may need to be able to split off the bad experiences from good ones and may be able to hold quite contradictory positions and ways of relating to the world. The recurrent employment of such defences early in life can lay down the tracks for the development of a particular kind of personality style or type. Without intervention or treatment (and even with these in some cases), children suffering from Type II Disorders may go on to develop adult personality disorders such as Dissociative Identity Disorder (or what was previously referred to as Multiple Personality Disorder) and Borderline Personality Disorder. Terr[33] also acknowledges that there may be situations in which Type I and II patterns overlap.

In the case of Type I Disorders, children are required to develop the means to integrate the experience of the trauma and to go forward in the world despite what has happened. Their energy is primarily expended in dealing with something that took place in the past, although their attempts to come to terms with the shock of a trauma will clearly affect their behaviour in the present. Terr suggests that four characteristics or symptoms are typical in most cases of childhood trauma. These include visualised or otherwise repeatedly perceived memories; repetitive behaviours; trauma-specific fears; and changed attitudes about people, life and the future.[34] It is apparent that some of these features could be understood as falling within the psychiatric diagnostic system of DSM IV-TR[35] discussed in Chapter 3. For example, repeatedly perceived memories would clearly fall under the intrusive or re-experiencing symptom cluster of PTSD and there are also overlaps with both avoidance and hyperarousal symptoms. The DSM system makes allowance for the classification of children within the category of PTSD, at points indicating that children's symptoms may present in a slightly different way, for example in repetitive play or disorganised behaviour,[36] but that they essentially parallel those of adult patients. In offering a clinically rich, observation-based overview of children's responses to trauma, Terr[37] paints a more elaborated picture of childhood trauma responses. She writes in such a way that we get a feel for what a child may be experiencing. For example, in discussing the case of a little girl who had undergone several surgeries to heal head wounds sustained when she was unexpectedly attacked by a circus lion, she describes how the girl would insist on playing hairdresser with her friends and how she would often hurt the younger children with the roughness of her brushing, seemingly trying to get rid of her feelings of fear and difference and indirectly expressing her anger at what had happened. Reading such case material brings home the importance of careful observation of traumatised children in order to understand the specific impact of the trauma for the child concerned.

In the case of children who have experienced single event traumas, Terr[38] also goes on to describe the fact that they often have very clear and vivid memories of the event, indeed sometimes better memories than adults (unlike Type II children whose memories may be vague). In younger children, as will be discussed in further detail, their difficulty in clearly distinguishing fantasy from reality and their 'egocentrism' or sense of their central place in their limited worlds, may lead them to seek explanations for bad events that are self-referenced and faulty in terms of logic. For example, a little girl of four who witnessed the drive-by shooting of her mother at a taxi terminus in Soweto on the way to take her to pre-school, was concerned that she may have caused her mother's death by feeling angry towards her following an argument over using the toilet before they left the house. She had linked her own aggression towards her mother with the later violence and was struggling to deal with feelings of guilt as well as fear, shock and loss. Terr[39] suggests that children may experience 'omens' or premonitions about events, have misperceptions that may even take the form of hallucinations on occasion, and may develop rituals to protect themselves. We see this in milder form in anxious children who need to check under their beds or in a cupboard before they go to sleep. Terr's work gives a rich picture of how children are affected by trauma that usefully complements the DSM formulation.

In some respects, discussing the way in which trauma affects children as a whole is somewhat misleading, as the term is used to include all those who might be considered minors or not yet adult in terms of society, in South Africa all those under the age of sixteen or eighteen years. In reading about children and trauma it is perhaps important to remember that adolescents, and more particularly those in late adolescence, may need to be understood as having characteristics of both adult and child responses. Another useful angle from which to discuss how trauma may present or show itself in children is to look at how children at varying stages of development in terms of the life cycle are differently affected.[40]

Developmental Differences in Trauma Presentations

Very young infants can be traumatised, although their ability to comprehend what has happened and express this is obviously limited. They may experience trauma primarily as pain when they have been physically hurt or as anxiety if they pick up distress or agitation in their caretakers. Children between the ages of zero and two years will tend to express distress primarily physically, such as through sleeping or eating difficulties. They may be more easily distressed, more irritable and more difficult to settle, but their response to trauma will be strongly dependent on how their caretakers respond to the trauma. A little girl of 2-years-old who was masturbated over by an uncle was roughly scrubbed in a very hot bath by her hysterical mother when she discovered the abuse. The child subsequently refused to eat solid foods, became aggressive towards her parents and preoccupied with touching her genital area. When her mother became calmer and was helped to manage her own distress through some counselling then the child's behaviour improved and her distress seemed to ease.

In early childhood, between the ages of about three and six years, children's lives are very focused on their homes and families. They are also at an age when their rational thinking capacity is not yet fully developed and they have rich fantasy lives. Children at this age, in accordance with Erikson's psychosocial theory of development,[41] are beginning to learn to do things for themselves, such as to dress and feed themselves. Exposure to trauma may compromise this development of autonomy, and traumatised young children may become clingy and dependent, returning to behaviour more in keeping with earlier stages of development. Their capacity for fantasy may mean that they also become fearful of imaginary dangers and young children often have nightmares linked to the trauma. As alluded to previously, their faulty logic sometimes leads them to hold themselves responsible for what took place or for what might take place in the future. A little boy of five who slept through an armed robbery in his home in which his older brother was injured, began to insist that he would not go to sleep unless his cricket bat was under his bed in case he needed to defend the family if the robbers came back again. Children of this age look to caretakers for reassurance and simple and clear explanations for events. Their fearfulness and increased dependence need to be accepted, certainly in the initial period following a trauma, after which they should be encouraged to gradually develop more confidence and independence again.

In middle childhood, from about seven to eleven years, a child's focus shifts to some extent away from home to the school context. Making relationships with other children and other adults, such as teachers, becomes important, as does formal learning. Children who experience trauma at this stage of development are better able to comprehend what has happened because of their more sophisticated thinking capacity. This can be helpful but can also lead to difficulties when it contributes to reality-based fear and disillusionment at such a young age. What is also evident is that traumatised children's concentration is affected and there is often deterioration in school performance and a tendency to be easily distracted.[42] Although less common, in some cases the opposite is true, and a child may become perfectionistic and highly achievement oriented, attempting to establish control and mastery in the part of their lives where they feel this is possible. Achieving well academically may be a way of defending against anxious, helpless and fearful emotions. Children may also struggle interpersonally, feeling now different from their peers and somewhat self-conscious. Like younger children, these junior school-aged children may also become more dependent and fearful of being left alone. Again it is important for caretakers to respond as openly as possible to the trauma and to help their child to talk about their experiences and fears in a sensitive and non-pressurising way. It may be important for the school to be made aware of what has happened and to look at how supports can be put in place without invasion of the child's privacy. In some instances group support for pupils may be helpful if the trauma has affected them as a collective. In a case in which a twelve year-old girl was shot on her way to school in Johannesburg as a bystander to an armed robbery, the school organised a peaceful march of pupils and parents and the collection of funds to assist with better policing. The principal reported that the children seemed to feel better to be able to do something active in response to their classmate's homicide.[43]

From the age of about twelve until eighteen years children move into the stage of adolescence, involving large physical, mental and social changes. The sense of being male or female is strengthened with body changes and there is an increased interest in sexual and partner relationships. It is almost a cliché that adolescents become very focused on and invested in the acceptance of their peer group and more challenging of their parents' attitudes and behaviours. With the development of formal operational thinking comes the capacity to think symbolically and to become more interested in political, philosophical and spiritual issues, although this tends to happen in later adolescence and young adulthood. Traumatisation in adolescence can take a number of paths. Some adolescents become withdrawn, uncommunicative and almost 'shut down'. Others become defiant, oppositional and even aggressive in their manner. Given the propensity for experimentation and risk-taking at this age, trauma may precipitate substance abuse and reckless behaviour. For many adolescents though, the central difficulty is in making sense of the event and what this means for their identity and their understanding of life values. Given that this is a strongly formative stage in terms of these dimensions, it is hoped that intervention can help an adolescent put the traumatic event into perspective without it necessarily leading to the setting of a negative life outlook. It may also be difficult to persuade adolescents to accept help or support as this may be viewed as compromising independence and they are often highly self-conscious in both individual and group therapy settings. Nevertheless, intervention from a trusted adult can often assist a teenager to negotiate the trauma in a more thoughtful way and to prevent the likelihood of a negative developmental trajectory.

At all developmental stages it is important to recognise the resources of the child, such as the capacity for imagination or the need to begin to define a personal value system, and to marshal these strengths in supporting children and adolescents through trauma. It is apparent that it is important to marry generic understandings of trauma impact with a developmental perspective in order to do justice to the way in which children of different ages and developmental stages are likely to respond. Although the individual developmental attributes of a child are important in determining how trauma manifests, it has also been demonstrated in numerous contexts that the environment in which the child is traumatised (be this family, immediate community or broader society), plays a significant role in outcomes.

Familial, Social and Community Dimensions

A common finding in trauma research with children, and one that makes intuitive sense, is that parents or caregivers play a crucial role in whether exposure to trauma leads to symptomatology or disorder, or whether the child recovers relatively unscathed from the event. If caretakers, particularly mothers, are traumatised themselves the likelihood of children manifesting distress in increased. While it is common for parents to experience their own distress and even some posttraumatic symptoms after their child has experienced a trauma, a very high level of parental distress can impede a parent's capacity to create a secure and predictable post-trauma environment for the child and to provide emotional containment for the child's fear and anxiety.[44] Several South African studies have found that there is a significant correlation between the presentation of symptoms in children and level of symptomatology reported by the mother.[45] Similarly, in a study conducted amongst Palestinian children exposed to military violence it was found that the group 'most vulnerable to intrusion symptoms were younger girls whose mothers showed high levels of PTSD symptoms'[46] and that high levels of avoidance symptoms were also strongly associated with mothers' PTSD symptoms. A study into the effects of the 9/11 attack in New York on a national sample of adolescents also found that their levels of posttraumatic stress symptoms were associated with parental distress, amongst other factors.[47] It seems that parental distress is generally a good predictor of child distress. This finding is in keeping with some psychoanalytic understandings of the impact of trauma that suggest that traumas represent attacks on attachment[48] and involve experiences of loss. In object relations terms it is suggested that the harm sustained during a trauma is experienced as a failure by good caretaking 'objects' (people or representations of people in an individual's life) to protect one in the face of danger. If one's primary caretaker (usually the object who is most strongly internalised to create a kind of an internal protective mechanism) is also clearly harmed by an experience, then there is likely to be increased anxiety on the part of a child. The sense that the world is a bad place full of harmful 'objects' and that good objects (in this case the mother or parents) are helpless in the face of such badness, is likely to increase distress, fear and despair. This is most particularly the case with younger children whose models of the world and relationships are still being developed. Such ideas would also resonate with those of Janoff-Bulman[49] concerning basic assumptions, discussed in Chapter 4. A child whose parents or caretakers seem overwhelmed and disorganised by a traumatic event is likely to be more vulnerable to questioning their beliefs about how benign and meaningful the world is.

It is important to recognise that family or caretaking systems do not exist in isolation and that community and societal stability, cohesion, values, resources and social capital, also play an important role in childhood trauma. Community psychology perspectives emphasise the importance of context in understanding both group and individual problems. To reiterate the premise touched on in the introduction, it is apparent that community upheaval and disruption, such as what takes place during both national and international conflicts and wars, not only places children at risk for victimisation and traumatisation but also compromises the recovery context. Referring to a UNICEF report in a book published in 1997, Rock writes, 'During the last 10 years alone, 2 million children have been killed, 4 to 5 million have been disabled, 12 million left homeless, and 10 million left psychologically traumatised. More than a million have been orphaned or separated from their parents'.[50] Since then there have been wars in Eastern Europe and Iraq, and in Africa there has been the war in the Democratic Republic of the Congo, ongoing conflict in Sudan and political battles in Kenya and Zimbabwe, amongst other instances of severe social upheaval. Thousands of children are impacted by these kinds of events. In addition, although not necessarily categorised as traumatic stressors in the classic sense, it is also apparent that poverty, political repression, gender oppression and various forms of discrimination create a climate for traumatisation. Butchart and colleagues[51] point out that amongst the victims of trauma the poor and oppressed are disproportionably represented. While recognising that it is impossible to do justice to this scale of 'social ills', two trauma-related sets of difficulties that illustrate the importance of community-level understandings will be briefly discussed – the issue of youth involvement in protest politics and the issue of AIDS-related parental bereavement.

Although South Africa has moved on markedly from the era of apartheid politics and the struggles associated with the implementation and contestation of a race- and class-based system of oppression, a large body of trauma work in South Africa was generated in response to this historical climate. At the time of the 1994 democratic elections the Goldstone Commission was set up to 'undertake an inquiry into the effects of public violence and intimidation on children'.[52] The findings of this commission are well documented in the final report but were also disseminated in a book entitled *Spirals of Suffering*.[53] Both texts provide telling accounts of the effects of the apartheid system and state repression on the lives of children. One group of children that received particular attention were those who became involved in protest politics and the armed struggle, the majority of these boys aged from twelve to eighteen years, but some even younger. These youth were subject to tear-gassing and arrest, detention without trial, torture, house arrest, forced re-education camp attendance and in some cases, were killed. For example, over 15,000 children were detained between the years of 1960 and 1994 and between 1984 and 1986 security force violence claimed the lives of 300 children and 18,000 were arrested on protest charges.[54] There is acknowledgement of the brutalising effect of the conflict and of the fact that for the youth involved in the struggle, the young 'comrades', the long-term effects of precocious engagement in violent conflict were difficult to gauge, but potentially harmful to them and others. Up until the present, children continue to be recruited into armed forces (in many African countries in particular) and there is ongoing concern about the identity of 'child soldiers' and what this means for their own and their societies' futures. Some of the long-term consequences of child and adolescent engagement in township paramilitary structures in South Africa in the early 1990s appear to be social alienation, substance use and some rigidity of identity for many of these boys who are now men.[55] When children are victims of structural violence in the kinds of large numbers suggested here it is clear that change needs to take place at structural and political levels and that individual treatment of trauma victims may be unfeasible and limited in efficacy.

A more contemporary, community-level, trauma-related problem in South Africa is that of loss of a parent or parents due to AIDS. While death of a parent due to illness might not always constitute a traumatic stressor (and, for older adults, is in the normal order of life), for children such a loss is often experienced as traumatic, even if anticipated. One of the central concerns arising out of Cluver and Gardner's[56] study of AIDS orphans cited previously, is that levels of traumatic stress amongst these children were very high. Although they are cautious not to over-generalise their findings, in part because of how levels of traumatic stress were assessed, they nevertheless conclude that the 'findings of strikingly high PTSD-type symptoms ... indicate that this should be a key area for research and intervention'.[57] They also propose that a number of aspects of AIDS-related bereavement may contribute to traumatisation. They write that 'many children witness the slow, painful death of a parent in degrading circumstances. The intermittent nature of the disease, stigma and secrecy around the death, the move into foster care, into a child-headed household, or onto the streets, could all potentially contribute to trauma for children'.[58] Thus there appear to be multiple features that are implicated in AIDS-related bereavement, including exposure to physically repugnant images (such as the abjection of a dying parent) and the social isolation stemming from ongoing shame and stigmatisation. This is clearly a kind of event that has multiple traumatic elements with both immediate and long-term impacts. Interestingly a recent study of AIDS-orphaned children in South Africa found strong evidence that perceived social support played an ameliorating role with regard to the rates of traumatic stress symptoms observed in a group of 425 children.[59] This study reinforces the idea that the impact of becoming orphaned due to AIDS-related death of a parent or parents is complex and multi-dimensional. The fact that social support appears to play a positive role in preventing the development of traumatic stress conditions suggests that both lack of stigmatisation and the active involvement of others in one's future survival may make a difference to vulnerable children. The study also points to the importance of social level interventions as will be discussed later. While this cursory coverage of AIDS-related bereavement cannot do justice to the complexity of the problem, it is apparent that this is a traumatic stressor that is affecting and will increasingly affect large numbers of children in South Africa. The scope of the problem again suggests that multi-level and multi-faceted intervention is required. In the same way that the impact of trauma needs to be understood at both individual and systemic levels, intervention in response to trauma also needs to be understood as involving many kinds of intervention which can be used in complementary ways.

Treating Childhood Trauma

Treating trauma in children can take place at a number of levels. These include: individual treatment for the child; parent or caretaker support and counselling; group psychotherapy; and community or organisational interventions, such as school-based projects.[60]

There is considerable overlap between the types of individual interventions used for adults and children, child treatment also encompassing debriefing and both short- and longer-term psychotherapy. Pharmacotherapy or drug treatment may also be used with children and adolescents but is still somewhat controversial as the effects of drug treatment on children have not been well enough established.[61] Psychotherapy approaches include cognitive behavioural therapy, psychodynamic psychotherapy, narrative and systemic interventions.[62] For children aged between about four and twelve years, play therapy is the most commonly used intervention, often employing drawing and creative activities and/or play with objects representing the trauma. One of the most widely cited brief term approaches is 'The child interview' developed by Pynoos and Eth[63] for child witnesses or victims of violent incidents. Although designed as a brief-term model for early intervention, it can be used to assist children to work through Type I traumas more generally. The model involves encouraging and supporting the child to recount their experiences and associated fears and then helping them to explore and process what has happened, giving particular attention to misperceptions, feelings of responsibility and self-blame and how the child is making sense of the event. The child client is assisted to 'work through' these issues and there is encouragement to take a future-oriented perspective and to look at ways of managing bad feelings if they recur. The model facilitates the processing of trauma using the common principles that guide most interventions with children: assisting the child to face and process the event; to gain some sense of understanding of what took place; and to regain some sense of control, trust and hope. Treatment also often involves identifying adults who the child can usefully call upon for assistance and helping the child to access such support so that there is containment beyond the therapy.

Particularly with very young children, but also with older children, psychoeducation of parents may be important in helping them to become more effective in their support.[64] Caretakers can offer ongoing care outside of a therapy setting and may be able to assist their children in day-to-day circumstances.[65] By supporting parents to manage their own feelings of distress and by giving them helpful input about what to anticipate and how best to respond to their child's needs, the therapist can create a context in which caretakers effectively become auxiliary counsellors. A case study documenting the use of this kind of approach in the treatment of a little girl from Alexandra township who had been raped illustrates how counselling of the mother enabled her to explore her child's experiences and feelings with greater confidence, and how this in turn helped the child to turn to her mother as a source of therapeutic support.[66] Assisting caretakers to become effective in helping their children to deal with their distress also restores a sense of safety and trust for the child and rebuilds or strengthens lasting relationships. This may sometimes require parallel therapy for parents and children when they have both been traumatised by events. For example, a mother and her twelve-year-old daughter who had lost their husband and father in a car accident seemed distant and conflicted in their first session together. It proved helpful to see them both separately for therapy for a period so that the mother could express her fear of single parent responsibility and the daughter her distress at losing the person she had perceived as her primary parent. It was only as the mother became less overwhelmed by grief and panic, having worked through her anxieties in therapy, that her daughter felt safer and began to share some of her own grief and adjustment difficulties with her surviving parent. Individual therapy seemed to create a transitional space for them to work through important issues in such a way that they were then able to engage more productively in some co-therapy before termination. The case study in Box 6.1 provides an account of both the presentation and treatment of a child trauma case illustrating many of the issues that have been highlighted thus far.

In some instances group interventions may be helpful. This is particularly the case when a group of children have all been affected by the same traumatic event, for example, in a school, club or social setting. Groups for children who have experienced the same kind of trauma (even when this occurred in unrelated settings) have also been found to be helpful, such as groups for refugee or HIV-positive children. Group interventions may involve creative forms of therapy such as drama, dance and art-making, as well as more conventional talk-based psychotherapy. An intervention of the latter kind took place at a girls' school where pupils away on a camp had been affected by a lightning strike, causing the death of one child and severe injury to two others. In addition to giving a talk to the whole school about the impact of trauma and bereavement, two therapists also ran an eight-session, semi-structured, discussion-based group for girls who had been on the camp

Box 6.1
Case study of an intervention with a traumatised child

Tulani, a little boy of five years, was brought to a trauma clinic in Johannesburg by his mother. She described how his behaviour had changed following a taxi accident some months previously. Initially she said he had seemed alright but now he was afraid to let her out of his sight and refused to travel in any kind of motorised transport. This created difficulties for her as it meant that she either had to walk to places with him or leave him behind when she travelled long distances, despite his crying and clinging to her when she left the house. She was planning to travel to Limpopo over a forthcoming long weekend and was concerned as to how she would manage Tulani's fears as she planned to take him with her to visit his grandmother. She also reported that his play-school teacher had noticed that he was more withdrawn and that he was asking for assistance with tasks that he had previously begun to manage on his own. For example, he asked her to cut up his food for him and would forget where he had put his school bag. She said that his concentration had also deteriorated and that he seemed to go into a kind of day-dream at times. Her younger brother who lived with them had also noticed changes and was trying to spend more time with his nephew.

In further discussion it emerged that Tulani and his mother had both been involved in the accident together when the taxi in which they were travelling swerved to avoid a pedestrian and overturned. Tulani sustained minor injuries in the form of a cut to his hand but his mother, who was thrown out of the vehicle, had hit her head and been unconscious for about 20 minutes. Together with some other passengers they had been taken to a hospital where, after examination, they were both discharged. The mother reported no further symptoms on her part, other than some occasional headaches. She said that it had been difficult to take taxi transport initially but that she was now used to this again and that such travel was necessary. She repeated her observation that Tulani had initially seemed fine and when questioned confirmed that he had not sustained any head or other injuries beyond the cut to his hand. She recalled that he had woken up crying on two or three occasions soon after the accident but that his sleep had then improved. Her main concern was his extreme fear of going near or travelling in any motor vehicle, a fear that seemed to have grown stronger with time. Although she was mostly sympathetic, there were times when she felt exasperated with him. Tulani himself was a shy boy and during the first session that he and his mother had with the therapist, he spoke very little on his own behalf. He seemed rather anxious but was also cooperative and endearing in his manner.

Tulani was treated over the course of ten weeks of therapy. It was decided that he and his mother should be offered separate interventions, with the mother receiving some personal counselling, psychoeducation and parental guidance, and Tulani receiving play therapy with a different therapist. It was suggested to the mother that it was her injury and apparent abandonment of Tulani at the very frightening time immediately after the accident that had been most difficult for him and with counselling she was able to better understand his fears. Tulani was initially quite shy and inhibited in the playroom and would only leave his mother when shown where he could find her if necessary. Over two sessions, however, he began to trust the therapist and seemed eager to go into the playroom. During his play therapy sessions he initially did some drawing but then concentrated on building roads in the sandpit and playing with cars that in many instances bumped and overturned. He seemed quite energised in playing this kind of game over and over. The therapist interpreted the possible parallels between his play and the trauma incident, focusing on his concerns about injury and need for reassurance. It appeared that at the time that his mother was unconscious he had feared that she was dead and had indeed struggled to comprehend what was happening. He emphasised the noise of the accident often in his play and it was clear that a sense of danger had become associated with loud noises. His later play became extended into acting out scenes in which people became injured and he would sometimes instruct the therapist that she was injured and offer to bandage parts of her body. He would also pretend to cook her food which they would share, seemingly indicating that he wanted to restore a sense of harmony in his life and that he perhaps had seen his mother as being in need of care. Again the play therapist made links between his fears during the accident and his attempts to make things better.

About four sessions into the therapy it was decided to add a behavioural component to the treatment in parallel with the play therapy. It was agreed that in the company of both the therapist and his mother (in keeping with the principles of systematic desensitisation) Tulani would be encouraged to begin to get used to motor cars again. On the first occasion, after some preparation from the therapist, Tulani, his mother and the play therapist all spent some time looking at and then just sitting in a car for a part of the session. On the next occasion all three were driven a short distance around the parking lot and the following week they drove once around the block in traffic. On each occasion Tulani's fears were acknowledged and he was reassured by both his mother and the therapist, being praised for his bravery in tackling something so difficult for him. He also chose to bring an action figure from the playroom with him which seemed to represent some courageous part of himself but was also seen as being protective of him. Although Tulani's mother wanted to increase the steps that he was taking after the first week, the importance of a gradual approach, allowing Tulani to overcome his fears and relax sufficiently at each stage, was explained to her. However, on their arrival at therapy after the third week of the behavioural treatment she reported that they had needed to take a taxi to do some shopping and that Tulani had come willingly with her after she had reassured him that they could get off the taxi if he became too frightened. They had successfully completed a round trip to the shopping centre and back and she was very excited. Tulani also seemed proud to report what he had achieved. After a couple more sessions allowing Tulani to consolidate his progress and to prepare for termination, the therapist and he had a farewell session and special tea to end the therapy. While Tulani found it difficult to say goodbye to the therapist, he and his mother seemed close and happier. The mother's involvement in both her own and his therapy indicated her level of commitment to the process and to her child and suggested that she would continue to support him after termination. The therapeutic team found the work with Tulani and his evident improvement very rewarding.

at the time. The girls were aged between about ten and twelve years so were able to verbalise their concerns within the group. Group work allows therapists to meet the needs of several children at a time and also often helps to de-stigmatise traumatic responses and promote interpersonal support. The local Wilderness therapy programmes developed by the National Peace Accord Trust[67] and the AIDS story book project[68] are two examples of how group work with children and youth can be innovative, embracing principles of both group psychotherapy and community intervention.

The findings of one South African study of the effects of community violence on children suggest that, while support from families and schools can moderate the impact of trauma, there is a limit to what these sources of social support can do to buffer the effects of community violence.[69] Ultimately, finding ways to reduce or prevent violence and trauma in the first instance is the most effective way to protect children from distress. Community-based interventions, which address traumatisation in even broader groups of children, frequently take the form of preventative rather than curative interventions. There are numerous school-based programmes that have been designed, for example, to tackle issues of violence prevention, sexual abuse/coercion and death and bereavement. Such interventions aim to prepare children to deal with difficult events as well as to avoid dangers and risks. There is some evidence that after-school activities played a role in reducing anxiety amongst early adolescents growing up in a high-violence area in Cape Town,[70] suggesting that even interventions of a more general nature (such as sporting, creative or social activities) may protect children against the worst impact of trauma exposure. However, when trauma has already taken place, community interventions are often helpful in providing symbolic as well as literal kinds of support to victims, for example, in the singing of songs, saying of prayers and construction of symbols of remembrance. The school march described earlier could be seen as such a kind of community intervention. Community interventions of this kind are often explicitly geared to create a sense of community cohesion and common humanity. In this respect they can assist in rebuilding positive meaning systems for children who have been traumatised as well as a sense of belonging to a containing social group.

Conclusion

Children who have been traumatised represent an important category of victims or survivors requiring acknowledgement and intervention. However, it may be useful to sound a word of caution in recognising that they are also a group of victims whose identity is open to exploitation. The idea of the innocent 'child victim' can be manipulated at times for political leverage and public recruitment around social agendas. The victimisation of children almost inevitably sparks particular civil outrage, as perhaps it should. It is important though, that in highlighting the plight of children for political ends intervention with the victims themselves does not take second place. In concluding this chapter on children and trauma it is perhaps useful to entertain a critical perspective and to think carefully about how child traumatisation is represented in the media and popular discourse[71] and what this might say about the perceived agency of children in general and about the legitimacy (or illegitimacy) of adult trauma survivors. As has been argued, children are vulnerable to traumatisation of a range of kinds and the impact of this in the form of psychological distress and psychiatric disorders has been well-documented. Both more classically psychotherapeutic and community-based interventions appear to be helpful in addressing trauma in children. Part of the prevention of future trauma lies in the treatment of those who are damaged as children since this may operate to curb ongoing cycles of violence brought about by the re-enactment of victim and victimiser positions. Child trauma intervention thus has potential benefits for both the individuals concerned and the broader society. The resilience and resourcefulness of children in overcoming trauma also needs to be foregrounded. In South Africa we need to hold the tension of recognising both the damage sustained and the extraordinary strengths displayed by children who are traumatised in multiple ways in this country.

Chapter 7

CONCLUSION

The psychoanalytic view of trauma argues that until traumatic experiences and their personal meaning are fully recognised, understood and 'owned' by the survivor, these experiences will continue to manifest themselves in symptoms of distress and unconscious re-enactments of the original traumatic situation. Perhaps this also provides a useful analogy for a traumatised society. Until we have a fuller understanding of the types of trauma that South Africans are exposed to, and the full range of the psychological impact of and meaning attached to such experiences, traumatisation in South African society is likely to be repeated from one generation to the next. An illustration of this possible kind of effect is the fact that one of the findings of a series of panel hearings on violence in Western Cape schools, held by the South African Human Rights Commission in 2006, was that children as young as seven frequently engage in games called 'rape me rape me' and 'hit me hit me' in the playground, demonstrating how endemic and normalised violence has become for the very young members of our society.[1]

Given what we know about the prevalence rates of different forms of direct and indirect trauma exposure in South African society, it should be no surprise that trauma is a common, even normal, part of the lives of many South Africans of all ages, including young children. But in order to really understand the psychological impact of this exposure, to be truly mindful of what it means to live in a context of chronic danger, the meaning and functions of behaviours such as playground games about violence need to be carefully explored. A layered psychological understanding might suggest a range of different possible meanings and functions of such playground enactments, including that they are a form of traumatic re-experiencing, an active attempt at mastery over situations that make children feel anxious, a way of trying to understand things they commonly see and hear about in their homes and community, or a form of identification with adults (developmentally parallel to the more benign games of 'house house' or 'doctor doctor' that many young children engage in to 'practice' adult roles). Such games may indeed be considered a symptom of posttraumatic stress; on the other hand, turning potentially frightening domestic or community events into a playground game may be an indication of children's resilience and capacity for coping in the face of endemic trauma. Without a fuller exploration of the meaning of such behaviours, we cannot really know exactly what they might mean for our youth and how best to engage with them and offer optimal support.

We would like to conclude this book by emphasising the need to continue to systematically document trauma exposure, impact and treatment in South African society in order to address important gaps in our knowledge and to continue to enhance our interventions, so that a legacy of trauma will not be passed on to future generations of South Africans. Throughout this book, we have described not only the state of knowledge about the prevalence, impact and treatment of trauma in the international literature, but also the many local knowledges that have emerged to date. In this chapter, we consider those local knowledges that remain to be documented, and suggest some ways forward.

We have seen in Chapter 2 that several different forms of trauma are extremely common in South Africa. Over the past fifteen years, endemic political violence has been replaced by high levels of criminal violence, intimate partner abuse, and physical and sexual assaults against women and children. Although South Africa does not necessarily have higher rates of all forms of violence than other countries, the severity

147

of violence in this country does appear to be particularly extreme – our rates of homicide and fatal sexual assaults are amongst the very highest in the world. In addition, many South Africans are traumatised by accidental injuries such as traffic accidents and burns. These direct forms of traumatisation are further compounded by indirect exposure to trauma, such as witnessing violence or hearing about the violent death of a loved one. It is therefore not surprising that the majority of South Africans have experienced not one but multiple traumas in their lives. Although no South Africans are entirely protected from trauma, it is apparent that South Africans of all ages who live in conditions of poverty are most at risk of experiencing many forms of violence and accidental injury.

In South Africa, as elsewhere, it is difficult to accurately establish the prevalence of certain forms of trauma, even with anonymous survey questionnaires. Sexual violence and coercion is probably under-reported and experiences of child abuse are hard to assess with younger children. And given that memory disturbances and avoidance of traumatic material are common psychological consequences of trauma, it must be assumed that trauma reporting in general is prone to inaccuracies. While bearing these issues in mind, we now have a number of prevalence studies, community studies, clinic studies and other valuable sources of data that contribute to an emerging picture of the scope and severity of trauma exposure in South Africa. What is less clear, however, is the psychological impact of trauma exposure in our society and the best ways in which to ameliorate this.

Compared with economically developed countries, there has been less published research on the psychological effects of trauma in economically developing countries. In South Africa too, the amount of published research on the psychological effects of trauma (as opposed to patterns of trauma exposure) is surprisingly small given the scope and scale of trauma exposure in our society and the amount of rich clinical experience that interventionists working with trauma survivors in a variety of settings have accumulated. As discussed in Chapter 3, where South African researchers have attempted to explore the impact of trauma, their approach to doing so has often been framed by research trends in economically developed countries, in particular the use of PTSD symptom scales to assess the impact of trauma exposure. While it is useful to have information about posttraumatic symptoms that can be compared across countries, there are some limitations to exploring the impact of trauma through the use of highly structured tools developed in contexts other than our own.

PTSD, comorbid disorders like depression, phobias and substance abuse, and complex PTSD (or Disorders of Extreme Stress) are trauma consequences that have been identified by clinicians and researchers in North America, Canada, the United Kingdom and European countries. Establishing how common they are in other contexts, and particularly in one that is as diverse with regard to language, culture and socio-economic circumstances as South Africa, is a complex matter indeed. In recent years, the relevance of the PTSD diagnostic category to non-'Western' cultures (that is, cultural contexts outside of the United States, the United Kingdom and Europe) has been debated.[2] This argument forms part of a broader debate regarding 'etic' and 'emic' processes in mental health research.[3] The term 'etic' refers to the process of applying a particular (usually 'Western') meaning system across all cultures. Studies that apply the PTSD diagnosis to cultures outside of the context in which it was developed, for example, by assessing PTSD symptoms using questionnaires or structured interviews for PTSD developed in the United States or the United Kingdom, are adopting an etic perspective on mental illness. By contrast, the term 'emic' refers to the exploration of culturally unique meaning systems. Studies applying emic principles attempt to understand the subjective meaning of the illness experience for the sufferer. This subjective experience is always culturally mediated – that is, it is patterned by, or filtered through the lens of, local cultural meaning systems.[4] This subjective 'insider' perspective can often best be accessed by asking people to describe in an open, unstructured way what they are experiencing and how they understand this, rather than by asking them to endorse an existing list of symptoms.

Some researchers are tempted to argue in favour of one approach over the other. For example, those who favour an etic approach could argue that certain biological and neurobiological processes involved in trauma responses (such as the body's fight-or-flight response) are universal and not culture-specific, or that researchers should use one standard tool (such as a PTSD questionnaire) to assess the occurrence of a psychiatric diagnosis in different contexts so that we can meaningfully compare the results. Those who favour an emic approach could argue that, by using a questionnaire to ask people whether or not they have symptoms that have been 'discovered' elsewhere, we could miss all those symptoms or experiences that do not fit neatly into these pre-defined categories. For example, a study with traumatised Sudanese refugees in Uganda and torture survivors in Malawi found that PTSD re-experiencing and hyperarousal symptoms were common in these samples, but that the classic avoidance symptoms of PTSD were rare.[5] Rather, avoidance appeared to be manifested through somatic symptoms of bodily numbing. As we noted in Chapter 3, a few local studies have similarly found that somatic symptoms are very common among South African trauma survivors. This suggests that, even when PTSD symptoms are present across different cultures, culture- and context-specific manifestations may be found if they are looked for. These local expressions of posttraumatic stress may require somewhat different interventions than those offered by mainstream trauma therapies. It is, therefore, apparent that both emic and etic approaches have something of value to offer, and that they should, in fact, supplement each other in order to develop a full understanding of traumatic stress in South Africa.

At this stage in the emergence of local knowledges about traumatic stress in South Africa, we would argue that the use of psychiatric tools from other countries should be just one of a range of methods for exploring the impact of trauma on the South African population, and that more qualitative research is needed to understand those aspects of trauma response that may be context-specific. However, when international tools are utilised, it is important that they be applied with clinical rigour. We saw in Chapter 3 that symptoms of posttraumatic stress certainly appear to be very common among South African trauma survivors in a wide variety of settings. However, the trend towards using self-report symptom scales, which do not allow one to establish with certainty the duration or impact of symptoms, makes it difficult to be certain whether these are transitory posttraumatic responses that fall within the normal range or whether they reflect the presence of PTSD. At the same time, we have also noted some emerging evidence to suggest that many trauma survivors in South Africa may suffer from non-specific forms of distress rather than from specific psychiatric disorders. Even when trauma survivors do not meet the clinical threshold for particular psychiatric diagnoses, it is, therefore, important that we document those psychological symptoms that do seem to persist in the aftermath of a trauma.

There are particular populations of trauma survivors in South Africa that require more careful and thorough understanding. Little has been documented locally regarding the impact of chronic abuse, either in childhood or in the context of intimate partner violence, even though some potentially useful diagnostic guidelines have emerged from other countries in the concepts of complex PTSD or Disorders of Extreme Stress. In other developing countries, there have been some attempts to assess the cross-cultural relevance of these concepts, with mixed results. While some of the symptoms associated with these syndromes (for example, difficulty with modulating anger) have been found in traumatised populations in Ethiopia, Algeria and Gaza, others (such as low self-esteem) have not.[6] But to date there has been little published research on these complex adaptations to prolonged abuse in South Africa, despite ample evidence of the high prevalence of both child abuse and intimate partner abuse in this country.

Survivors of rape, too, are generally surprisingly under-represented in existing South African studies. Although survivors of gender-based violence are often difficult to access as research participants, these methodological difficulties alone cannot account for the scarcity of systematic research on the psychological effects of rape in South Africa. Given the prevalence of rape in this country, and the finding that South African rape survivors are at higher risk for developing PTSD than survivors of many other forms of violence[7], it might be fruitful for South African researchers to reflect on other possible reasons for these silences and to begin to address this relatively neglected area more actively.

Chapter 6 highlighted the ways in which trauma presents differently in children of different ages and developmental stages. Although there have been a number of studies conducted with South African children and adolescents, these too have focused primarily on assessing symptoms of PTSD and depression rather than exploring developmentally specific manifestations of trauma. The findings of the report of the Human Rights Commission on school violence, noted earlier in this chapter, highlights the importance of developing local knowledges and understandings of the impact of trauma on our children and youth.

We saw in Chapter 2 that there is evidence that multiple trauma is extremely common in South Africa. At present there is little published research that has specifically explored the psychological consequences of multiple or continuous trauma in South Africa, or the ways in which poverty may impact on coping in circumstances of continuous trauma. Indeed, poverty, HIV/AIDS and chronic trauma exposure present a multiple burden to many South Africans.[8] This includes children who, as discussed in Chapter 6, must often cope with the loss of their parents to HIV/AIDS, surviving in conditions of poverty, and ongoing exposure to many different types of trauma. In a context of continuous traumatisation, it is possible that specific traumatic events may not stand out for a person as being particularly stressful or significant, but may rather be viewed as yet another challenge in the ongoing struggle for survival.[9] In one of the few qualitative studies with South African trauma survivors conducted to date,[10] PTSD symptoms were found to be present, but other concerns were more pressing, including somatic complaints and a prevailing sense of economic and political marginalisation. In other words, events that meet the definition of trauma provided by the DSM may not necessarily be afforded any more importance in people's minds than the stressors associated with meeting their basic survival needs (such as food, shelter and employment) and with chronic feelings of disempowerment. Some authors have argued that, in trying to capture the psychological impact of trauma, we cannot divorce the impact of specific traumatic events from the impact of ongoing structural violence in the form of extreme poverty and socio-economic disempowerment.[11]

In Chapter 4 we noted that some trauma research in other countries has extended beyond a focus on psychiatric symptoms to explore the role of meaning-making in adaptation to trauma. Even when psychiatric symptoms are absent, the impact of trauma on our fundamental beliefs about ourselves, others and the world can create significant and ongoing distress, anxiety and feelings of vulnerability. Alternatively, trauma can sometimes be a catalyst for psychological growth. With a few exceptions, the area of meaning-making has seldom been explored with South African trauma survivors. Since adaptation to trauma has so often been defined in the psychological literature as a struggle with meaning, and since meaning-making is patterned by culture and context, this seems an important avenue for South African researchers to explore. At the same time, it is important to recognise that the development of meaning after trauma requires a post-trauma space in which to reflect on and evaluate the trauma experience, a privilege that is denied to the many South Africans who live in contexts of ongoing trauma.

South African researchers are certainly not alone in focusing more on post-trauma pathology than on resilience – this trend is characteristic of the international trauma literature. However, the unfortunately high levels of trauma in South African society present us with an opportunity to better understand resilience and coping in contexts of frequent, multiple trauma. There is perhaps an opportunity for South Africans to offer some new insights on trauma resilience and coping among adults and children, rather than waiting for researchers in other countries to lead the way in this area.

As reviewed in Chapter 5, there are several intervention approaches developed in other countries that have been found to be effective for trauma survivors. In South Africa, those working with trauma survivors in a variety of settings have drawn on these existing models and adapted them, where necessary, to local needs and resources. However, trauma interventionists in this country continue to face many challenges, including the difficulty with accessing treatment for many people living in conditions of poverty, ongoing community violence which makes it difficult to establish the client's basic safety before proceeding with an exploration of past traumatic experiences, and the need to remain constantly aware of, and sensitive to, issues of cultural, racial, linguistic and class differences between therapists and clients. The development and evaluation of accessible, short-term, and culturally or contextually meaningful trauma interventions is an ongoing task. Finally, in exploring ways to assist trauma survivors, we need to look beyond individual treatment to ways of harnessing community support and resilience, and to re-conceptualise trauma intervention more holistically as an inter-disciplinary enterprise that involves not only mental health workers, but also non-governmental organisations in the community development sector and the state education, security, justice and social welfare systems, amongst others.

This book has attempted to present a comprehensive picture of the current state of knowledge about traumatic stress, both internationally and in South Africa, and to highlight issues that still require fuller understanding. While a solid local database of the effects of trauma on South Africans of all ages has begun to emerge, and some contextually responsive local adaptations of trauma intervention models have been developed, some important gaps in our knowledge remain. Two issues bear repeating. Firstly, while we need to be cognisant of international findings about trauma, we also need to continue to allow local, contextually-specific understandings and interventions to emerge. Secondly, the intersection of continuous trauma and the structural violence of poverty creates a particular challenge for South Africans that needs to be better understood. While legislated apartheid is a thing of the past, it is apparent that the burden of trauma and violence in South Africa is primarily borne by those groups and communities who are most socio-economically disempowered. We noted in Chapter 1 that the development of local knowledge about trauma has its early roots in the activist agenda of the apartheid era, and would like to conclude this book by emphasising that trauma researchers and practitioners in South Africa continue to have an important role as social activists. The careful documentation of emerging understandings about trauma exposure, impact, intervention and recovery is an important part of this role. We need to draw on the variety of experiences and resources we have as a society to join together in reducing trauma causative events, addressing the multiple needs of trauma survivors and bolstering our individual and communal resilience.

ENDNOTES

Chapter 1

1. Wilson, J. P. 1994. 'The historical evolution of PTSD diagnostic criteria: from Freud to DSM-IV'. *Journal of Traumatic Stress*, 7(3): 681–698.

2. Herman, J. 1992. *Trauma and recovery: the aftermath of violence from domestic abuse to political terror.* London: Basic Books, quote on page 9.

3. American Psychiatric Association 2000. *Diagnostic and statistical manual of mental disorders.* (4th edition, text revision). Washington DC: American Psychiatric Association.

Chapter 2

1. Williams, S. L., Williams, D. R., Stein, D. J., Seedat, S., Jackson, P. B. & Moomal, H. 2007. 'Multiple traumatic events and psychological distress: The South Africa Stress and Health Study.' *Journal of Traumatic Stress*, 20(5): 845–55.

2. Williams, D. R., Herman, A., Kessler, R. C., Sonnega, J., Seedat, S., Stein, D. J. et al. 2004. 'The South Africa Stress and Health Study: rationale and design'. *Metabolic Brain Disease*, 19: 135–47.

3. Amnesty International. 2007. *Annual report 2007.* London: Amnesty International Publications.

4. Truth and Reconciliation Commission. 1998. *Truth and Reconciliation Commission of South Africa report, Vol. 3.* Cape Town: CTP.

5. Although the authors reject the use of racially constructed terms as discriminatory, it is nevertheless necessary to use these terms insofar as they reflect the racialised nature of the oppression perpetrated by the South African state under the apartheid system. The term 'black South Africans' here refers to South Africans who were categorised by the Population Registration Act during apartheid as 'African', 'coloured', 'Asian' or 'Indian'.

6. Coleman, M. 1998. *A crime against humanity: analysing the repression of the apartheid state.* Johannesburg: Human Rights Commission.
7. TRC, 1998, vol. 3.
8. Ibid.
9. Kaminer, D., Grimsrud, A., Myer, L., Stein, D. & Williams, D. R. 2008. 'Risk for posttraumatic stress disorder associated with different forms of interpersonal violence in South Africa.' *Social Science and Medicine*, 67: 1589–95.
10. TRC, 1998, vol. 3
11. Ibid.
12. Kaminer et al., 2008.
13. Truth and Reconciliation Commission. 1998. *Truth and Reconciliation Commission of South Africa report, Vol. 1.* Cape Town: CTP.
14. See CSVR website, http//:www.csvr.org.za
15. Gear, S. 2002. *Wishing us away: challenges facing ex-combatants in the 'new' South Africa.* Violence and Transition Series, 8. Johannesburg: Centre for the Study of Violence and Reconciliation.
16. Altbeker, A. 2007. *A country at war with itself: South Africa's crisis of crime.* Johannesburg: Jonathan Ball, quote on page 12.
17. Seedat, M., Van Niekerk, A., Jewkes, R., Suffla, S. & Ratele, K. 2009. 'Violence and injuries in South Africa: prioritising an agenda for prevention.' *Lancet Special Issue: Health in South Africa*, August 2009: 68–79.
18. Altbeker, 2007.
    Shaw, M. 2002. *Crime and policing in post-apartheid South Africa: transformation under fire.* London: Hurst and Co.
19. Matzopoulos, R., Norman, R. & Bradshaw, D. (2004). 'The burden of injury in South Africa: fatal injury trends and international comparisons.' In S. Suffla, A. Van Niekerk & N. Duncan. (eds). *Crime, violence and injury prevention in South Africa: developments and challenges*, pp. 9–21. Tygerberg: Medical Research Council-University of South Africa Crime, Violence and Injury Lead Programme.
20. Altbeker, 2007.
21. Kaminer et al., 2008.
22. Norman, R., Matzopolous, R., Groenwald, P. & Bradshaw, D. 2007. 'The high burden of injuries in South Africa.' *Bulletin of the World Health Organisation*, 85: 695–702.
23. Kessler, R. C., Sonnega, A., Bromet, E., Hughes, M. & Nelson, C. B. 1995. 'Posttraumatic stress disorder in the National Comorbidity Survey.' *Archives of General Psychiatry*, 52(12): 1048–1060.
    Breslau, N., Kessler, R. C., Chilcoat H. D., Schultz, L. R., Davis, G. C. & Andreski, P. 1998. 'Trauma and posttraumatic stress disorder in the community: The 1996 Detroit Area Survey of Trauma.' *Archives of General Psychiatry*, 55(7): 626–32.

Stein, M., Walker, J., Hazen, A. & Forde, D. 1997. 'Full and partial posttraumatic stress disorder: findings from a community survey.' *American Journal of Psychiatry*, 154: 1114–19.

Norris, F. H., Murphy, A. D. Baker, C. K., Perilla, J. L., Gutierrez Rodriguez, F. & Gutierrez Rodriguez, J. 2003. 'Epidemiology of trauma and posttraumatic stress disorder in Mexico.' *Journal of Abnormal Psychology*, 112(4): 646–56.

24. Standing A. 2005. *The threats of gangs and anti-gangs policy: policy discussion paper.* Institute for Security Studies: Pretoria.

Steinberg, J. 2004. *The number.* Jonathan Ball: Johannesburg.

25. Ratele, K., Swart, L. & Seedat, M. 2009. 'Night-time fatal violence in South Africa.' In P. Hadfield (ed). *Nightlife and crime: social order and governance in international perspective*, pp. 277–93. London: Oxford University Press.

26. Seedat et al., 2009.

27. Masuku, S. 2002. 'Prevention is better than cure.' *SA Crime Quarterly*, 2: 1–7.

Burrows, S., Bowman, B., Matzopoulus, R. & Van Niekerk, A. 2001. *A profile of fatal injuries in South Africa 2000. Second Annual Report of the National Injury Mortality Surveillance System.* Tygerberg: Medical Research Council.

28. Williams et al., 2007.

29. Breslau, N. 2002. 'Epidemiologic studies of trauma, posttraumatic stress disorder and other psychiatric disorders.' *Canadian Journal of Psychiatry*, 47(10): 923–9.

30. Williams et al., 2007.

31. Seedat, S., van Noord, E., Vythilingum, B., Stein D. & Kaminer, D. 2000. 'School survey of exposure to violence and posttraumatic stress symptoms in adolescents.' *South African Journal of Child and Adolescent Mental Health*, 12(1): 38–44.

32. Burton, P. 2006. 'Easy prey: results of the national youth victimisation study.' *SA Crime Quarterly*, 16: 1–6.

33. Ibid.

34. Jewkes, R. & Abrahams, N. 2002. 'The epidemiology of rape and sexual coercion in South Africa: an overview.' *Social Science and Medicine*, 55(7): 1231–244.

Rasool, S., Vermaak, K., Pharoah, R., Louw, A. & Stavrou, A. 2002. *Violence against women: a national survey.* Pretoria: Institute for Security Studies.

35. Ludsin, H. & Vetten, L. 2005. *Spiral of entrapment: abused women in conflict with the law.* Johannesburg: Jacana Media.

36. Abrahams, N., Martin, L. J. & Vetten, L. 2004. 'An overview of gender-based violence in South Africa and South African responses.' In S. Suffla, A. Van Niekerk & N. Duncan (eds). *Crime, violence and injury prevention in South Africa: developments and challenges*, pp. 40–64. Tygerberg: Medical Research Council-University of South Africa Crime, Violence and Injury Lead Programme.

37. Heise, L., Ellsberg, M. & Gottemoeller, M. 1999. *Ending violence against women*. Baltimore: The John Hopkins University School of Public Health.
38. Kaminer et al., 2008.
39. Department of Health (DoH). 2002. *South Africa Demographic and Health Survey 1998: Final Report*. Pretoria: Department of Health.
40. Gupta, J., Silverman, J. G., Hemenway, D., Acevedo-Garcia, D., Stein, D. J. & Williams, D. R. 2008. 'Physical violence against intimate partners and related exposures to violence among South African men.' *CMAJ*, 179(6): 535–41.
41. DoH, 2002.
42. Jewkes, R., Penn-Kekana, L., Levin, J., Ratsaka, M. & Schreiber, M. 2001. 'Prevalence of emotional, physical and sexual abuse of women in three South African provinces.' *South African Medical Journal*, 91(5): 421–8.
43. Dunkle, K. L., Jewkes, R. K., Brown, H. C., Gray, G. E., McIntyre, J. A. & Harlow, S. D. 2004. 'Gender-based violence, relationship power, and risk of HIV infection in women attending antenatal clinics in South Africa.' *Lancet*, 363(9419): 1415–21.
44. Artz, L. 1999. *Violence against women in rural Southern Cape: exploring access to justice through a feminist jurisprudence framework*. Cape Town: Institute of Criminology, University of Cape Town.
45. Abrahams, N., Jewkes, R., Laubscher, R. & Hoffman, M. 2006. 'Intimate partner violence: prevalence and risk factors for men in Cape Town, South Africa.' *Violence and Victims*, 21(2): 247–64.
46. Dunkle, K. L., Jewkes, R. K., Nduna, M., Levin, J., Jama, N., Khuzwayo, N. et al. 2006. 'Perpetration of partner violence and HIV risk behaviour among young men in the rural Eastern Cape, South Africa.' *AIDS*, 20(16): 2107–14.
47. Seedat et al., 2009.
48. Human Rights Watch. 1995. *Violence against women in South Africa: state response to domestic violence and rape*. New York/Washington: Human Rights Watch.
49. Bollen, S., Artz, L., Vetten, L. & Louw, A. 1999. *Violence against women in metropolitan South Africa: a study on impact and service delivery* (Monograph No. 41). Johannesburg: Institute for Security Studies.
50. Creamer, M., Burgess, P. & McFarlane, A.C. 2001. 'Post-traumatic stress disorder: findings from the Australian National Survey of Mental Health and Well-being.' *Psychological Medicine*, 31: 1237–47.
Norris et al., 2003.
Zlotnick, C., Johnson, J., Kohn, R., Vicente, B., Rioseco, P. & Saldivia, S. 2006. 'Epidemiology of trauma, post-traumatic stress disorder (PTSD) and co-morbid disorders in Chile.' *Psychological Medicine*, 36: 1523–33.

51. Kessler et al., 1995.
 Stein et al., 1997.
52. Kaminer et al., 2008.
53. Creamer et al., 2001.
 Kessler et al., 1995.
 Norris et al., 2003.
54. Dunkle et al., 2004.
55. Martin, L. 1999. 'Violence against women: an analysis of the epidemiology and patterns of injury in rape homicide in Cape Town and in rape in Johannesburg.' Unpublished Masters dissertation. University of Cape Town, Cape Town.
56. See RAPCAN website, http//:www.rapcan.org.za/articles.htm
57. Finkelhor, D. & Jones, L. (2006). 'Why have child maltreatment and child victimization declined?' *Journal of Social Issues*, 62(4): 685–716.
58. DoH., 2002.
59. Jewkes et al., 2001.
60. Seedat et al., 2000.
61. Madu, S. N. & Peltzer, K. (2000). 'Risk factors and child sexual abuse among secondary school students in the Northern Province (South Africa).' *Child Abuse and Neglect*, 24(2): 259–68.
62. Buga, G. A. B., Amoko, D. H. A. & Ncayiyana, D. 1996. 'Sexual behaviour, contraceptive practices and reproductive health among school adolescents in rural Transkei.' *South African Medical Journal*, 86(5): 523–7.
63. Richter, L. 1996. *A survey of reproductive health issues among urban black youth in South Africa: final grant report*. Pretoria: Medical Research Council.
64. Collings, S. J. 1997. 'Child sexual abuse in a sample of South African women students: prevalence, characteristics and long-term effects.' *South African Journal of Psychology*, 27(1): 37–42.
 Madu, S. N. 2001. 'The prevalence and patterns of childhood sexual abuse and victim-perpetrator relationship among a sample of university students.' *South African Journal of Psychology*, 31(4): 32–7.
65. Finkelhor, D. 1994. 'Current information on the scope and nature of child sexual abuse.' *The Future of Children*, 4(2): 31–53.
66. Jewkes, R., Levin, J., Mbananga, N. & Bradshaw, D. 2002. 'Rape of girls in South Africa.' *Lancet*, 359(9303): 319–20.
67. Kaminer et al., 2008
68. Collings, S. J. 1995. 'The long-term effects of contact and non-contact forms of child sexual abuse in a sample of university men.' *Child Abuse and Neglect*, 19(1): 1–6.
 Madu et al., 2001.
 Madu & Peltzer. 2000.

69. Collings, S. J. 2005. 'Sexual abuse of boys in KwaZulu-Natal South Africa: a hospital-based study.' *Journal of Child and Adolescent Mental Health*, 17(1): 23–5.

70. Jewkes, R., Sikweyiya, Y., Morrell, R. & Dunkle, K. 2009. *Understanding men's health and use of violence: interface of rape and HIV in South Africa.* Tygerberg: Medical Research Council Gender and Health Research Unit.

71. Jewkes & Abrahams, 2002.

72. Jewkes at al., 2009.

73. Abrahams, N., Jewkes, R., Martin, L. J., Mathews, S., Vetten, L. & Lombard, C. 2009. 'Mortality of women from intimate partner violence in South Africa: a national epidemiological study.' *Violence and Victims*, 24(4): 546–56.

74. Martin, 1999.

75. Abrahams, N., Martin, L. J., Jewkes, R., Mathews, S., Vetten, L. & Lombard, C. 2008. 'The epidemiology and the pathology of rape homicide in South Africa.' *Forensic Science International*, 178: 132–8.

76. Swart, L., Gilchrist, A., Butchard, A., Seedat, M. & Martin, L. 1999. *Rape surveillance through district surgeons offices in Johannesburg, 1996–1998: evaluation and prevention implications.* Pretoria: Institute of Social and Health Sciences, University of South Africa.

77. Mgoqi, N. C. 2006. 'The role of assault severity, sex role beliefs, personality factors, attribution style and psychological impact in predicting coping with rape victimization.' Unpublished doctoral dissertation. University of the Witwatersrand, Johannesburg.

78. Kaminer et al., 2008.

79. Kessler et al., 1995.

80. Wauchope, B. A. & Strauss, M. A. 1990. 'Physical punishment and physical abuse of American children: incidence rates by age, gender and occupational class.' In M. A. Strauss & R. J. Gelles (eds). *Physical violence in American families*, pp. 133–48. New Brunswick, NJ: Transaction Publishers.

81. Kaminer et al., 2008.

82. Dawes, A., Long, W., Alexander, L. & Ward, C. L. 2006. *A situation analysis of children affected by maltreatment and violence in the Western Cape. A case report for the Research Directorate, Department of Social Services and Poverty Alleviation: Provincial Government of the Western Cape.* Cape Town: Human Sciences Research Council.

83. Matzopolous et al., 2004.

84. Ibid.

85. Sukhai, A., Noah, M. & Prinsloo, M. 2004. 'Road traffic injury in South Africa: an epidemiological overview for 2001.' In S. Suffla, A. Van Niekerk & N. Duncan (eds). *Crime, violence and injury prevention in South Africa: developments and challenges*, pp. 114–27. Tygerberg: Medical Research Council-University of South Africa Crime, Violence and Injury Lead Programme.

86. See Arrive Alive website, http//:www.arrivealive.co.za.

87. Williams et al., 2007

88. Bradshaw, D., Groenewald, P., Laubscher, R., Nannan, N., Nojilana, B. & Norman, R. 2003. *Initial burden of disease estimates for South Africa, 2000.* Tygerberg: Medical Research Council.

89. Matzopolous et al., 2004.

90. Van Niekerk, A., du Toit, N., Nowell, M. J., Moore, S. & Van As, A. B. 2004. 'Childhood burn injury: epidemiological, management and emerging injury prevention studies.' In S. Suffla, A. Van Niekerk & N. Duncan (eds). *Crime, violence and injury prevention in South Africa: developments and challenges,* pp. 145–57. Tygerberg: Medical Research Council-University of South Africa Crime, Violence and Injury Lead Programme.

91. Van Niekerk, A., Rode, H. & Laflamme, L. 2004. 'Incidence and patterns of childhood burn injuries in the Western Cape, South Africa.' *Burns,* 30: 341–7.

92. Ibid.

93. Kessler et al., 1995.
    Stein et al., 1997.

94. American Psychiatric Association, 2000.

95. Breslau et al., 1998.

96. Williams et al., 2007.

97. Kessler et al., 1995.
    Stein et al., 1997.
    Creamer et al., 2001.
    Norris et al., 2003.

98. Williams et al., 2007.

99. Ibid.

100. Kessler et al., 1995.
     Stein et al., 1997.
     Norris et al., 2003.

101. Martin, L. & Kagee, A. 2008. 'Lifetime and HIV-related PTSD amongst persons recently diagnosed with HIV.' *AIDS and Behavior* (consulted on 12 December 2008).
     Olley, B., Seedat. S. & Stein, D. J. 2006. 'Persistence of psychiatric disorders in a cohort of HIV/AIDS patients in South Africa: a 6-month follow-up study.' *Journal of Psychosomatic Research,* 61(4): 479–84.

102. Maiden, R. & Terreblanche-Lourens, P. 2006. 'Managing the trauma of community violence and workplace accidents in South Africa.' *Journal of Workplace Behavioral Health,* 21(3/4): 89–100.

103. MacNair, R. M. 2002. 'Perpetration-induced traumatic stress in combat veterans.' *Peace and Conflict: Journal of Peace Psychology,* 8: 63–72.

Stein, D. J., Williams, S. L., Jackson, P. B. Seedat, S., Myer, L., Herman, A. et al. 2009. 'Perpetration of gross human rights violations in South Africa: association with psychiatric disorders.' *South African Medical Journal*, 99(5 Pt 2): 390–5.

104. Seedat et al., 2009.

Chapter 3

1.   American Psychiatric Association. 2000. *Diagnostic and statistical manual of mental disorders* (4th ed., text revision). Washington DC: APA.

2.   O'Brien, L. S. 1998. *Traumatic events and mental health*. Cambridge: Cambridge University Press.

3.   Kilpatrick, D. G., Resnick, H. S., Freedy, J. R., Pelcovitz, D., Resick, P. A. & Roth, S. 1998. 'The posttraumatic stress disorder field trial: evaluation of the PTSD construct - criteria A through E.' In T. Widiger, A. Frances, H. Pincus, R. Ross, M. B. First & W. W. Davis (eds). *DSM-IV sourcebook, Vol. 4*, pp. 803–44. Washington, DC: American Psychiatric Association Press.

4.   Herman, J. L. 1992. *Trauma and recovery: from domestic abuse to political terror*. London: Pandora.

5.   Stein, D., Cloitre, M., Nemeroff, C. B., Nutt, D. J., Seedat, S., Shalev, A. et al. 2009. 'Cape Town consensus on posttraumatic stress disorder.' *CNS Spectrums*, 14(1): 52–58.

6.   Yehuda, R. 2000. 'Neuroendocrinology.' In D. Nutt, J. R. T. Davidson & J. Zohar (eds). *Post-traumatic stress disorder: diagnosis, management and treatment*, pp. 53–68. London: Martin Dunitz.

7.   American Psychiatric Association, 2000.
     Kessler, R. C., Sonnega, A., Bromet, E., Hughes, M. & Nelson, C. B. 1995. 'Posttraumatic stress disorder in the National Comorbidity Survey.' *Archives of General Psychiatry*, 52(12): 1048–60.

8.   American Psychiatric Association, 2000.

9.   Breslau, N. 1998. 'Epidemiology of trauma and posttraumatic stress disorder.' In R. Yehuda (ed.). *Review of psychiatry, Vol. 17*, pp. 1–30. Washington, DC: American Psychiatric Association.

10. Freud, S. 1920/1948. *Beyond the pleasure principle*. London: Hogarth Press and Janet, P. 1919/1925. *Psychological healing, Vol. 1*. Trans. E. Paul and C. Paul. New York: Macmillan.

11. Piaget, J. & Inhelder, B. 1969. *The psychology of the child*. New York: Basic.

12. Horowitz, M. S. 1992. *Stress response syndromes*. Northvale, N. J.: Jason Aronson, and Wigren, J. 1994. 'Narrative completion in the treatment of trauma.' *Psychotherapy*, 31(3): 415–23.

13. Piaget, J. 1962. *Play, dreams and imitation in childhood.* New York: Norton.
14. Van der Kolk, B. A. 1996*a*. 'Trauma and memory.' In B. A. van der Kolk, A. C. McFarlane & L. Weisaeth (eds). *Traumatic stress: the effects of overwhelming experience on mind, body and society,* pp. 279–302. New York: Guilford Press.
15. Breslau et al., 1998.
    Creamer, M., Burgess, P. & McFarlane, A. C. 2001. 'Post-traumatic stress disorder: findings from the Australian National Survey of Mental Health and Well-being.' *Psychological Medicine,* 31, 1237–47.
    Kessler et al., 1995
    Norris, F. H., Murphy, A. D. Baker, C. K., Perilla, J. L., Gutierrez Rodriguez F. & Gutierrez Rodriguez, J. 2003. 'Epidemiology of trauma and posttraumatic stress disorder in Mexico.' *Journal of Abnormal Psychology,* 112(4): 646–56.
16. Kaminer, D., Grimsrud, A., Myer, L., Stein, D. & Williams, D. R. 2008. 'Risk for posttraumatic stress disorder associated with different forms of interpersonal violence in South Africa.' *Social Science and Medicine,* 67: 1589–95.
17. Breslau et al., 1998.
    Kessler et al., 1995
    Norris et al., 2003.
    Stein, M., Walker, J., Hazen, A. & Forde, D. 1997. 'Full and partial posttraumatic stress disorder: findings from a community survey.' *American Journal of Psychiatry,* 154: 1114–9.
    Zlotnick, C., Johnson, J., Kohn, R., Vicente, B., Rioseco, P. & Saldivia, S. 2006. 'Epidemiology of trauma, post-traumatic stress disorder (PTSD) and co-morbid disorders in Chile.' *Psychological Medicine,* 36: 1523–33.
18. Breslau et al., 1998.
19. Kaminer, D. & Seedat, S. 2005. 'Posttraumatic stress disorder.' In S. Romans and M.V. Seeman (eds). *Women's mental health: a life-cycle approach,* pp.221–36. Baltimore: Lippincott, Williams and Wilkins.
20. Stein, D., Seedat, S., Herman, A., Moomal, H., Heeringa, S. G., Kessler, R. C. et al. 2008. 'Lifetime prevalence of psychiatric disorders in South Africa.' *British Journal of Psychiatry,* 192: 112–7.
21. Creamer et al., 2001.
22. Van der Kolk, 1996*a*.
23. Yehuda, R. 1999. 'Biological factors associated with susceptibility to posttraumatic stress disorder.' *Canadian Journal of Psychiatry,* 44(1): 21–32.
24. True, W. R., Rise, J., Eisen, S., Heath, A. C., Goldberg, J., Lyons, M. et al. 1993. 'A twin study of genetic and environmental contributions to liability for posttraumatic stress symptoms.' *Archives of General Psychiatry,* 50: 257–64.
25. Pitman, R. K., Gilbertson, M. W., Gurvits, T. V., May, F. S., Lasko, N. B., Metzger, L. J. et al. 2006. 'Clarifying the origin of biological abnormalities in PTSD through the study of identical twins discordant for combat exposure.' *Annals of the New York Academy of Sciences,* 1071: 242–54.

26. Brewin, C. R., Andrews, B. & Valentine, J. D. 2000. 'Meta-analysis of risk factors for posttraumatic stress disorder in trauma-exposed adults.' *Journal of Consulting and Clinical Psychology*, 68(5): 748–66.

27. Bonanno, G. A., Galea, S. Bucciarelli, A. & Vlahov, D. 2007. 'What predicts psychological resilience after disaster? The role of demographics, resources and life stress.' *Journal of Consulting and Clinical Psychology*, 75(5): 671–82, Brewin et al., 2000.

28. Andrews, B., Brewin, C. R., & Rose, S. 2003. 'Gender, social support and PTSD in victims of violent crime.' *Journal of Traumatic Stress*, 16: 421–7.

29. Guay, S., Billette, V. & Marchand, A. 2006. 'Exploring the links between posttraumatic stress disorder and social support: processes and potential research avenues.' *Journal of Traumatic Stress*, 19(3): 327–38.

30. Kimerling, R. & Calhoun, K. S. 1994. 'Somatic symptoms, social support, and treatment seeking among sexual assault victims.' *Journal of Consulting and Clinical Psychology*, 62: 333–40.

31. Esprey, Y. 1996. ' Post-traumatic stress and dimensions of trauma.' Unpublished Masters dissertation. University of the Witwatersrand, Johannesburg.

32. Williams, R. & Joseph, S. 1999. 'Conclusions: an integrative psychosocial model of PTSD.' In W. Yule (ed.). *Post-traumatic stress disorders: concepts and therapy*, pp. 297–314. Chichester, England: Wiley.

33. Brewin, C. R., MacCarthy, B. & Furnham, A. 1989. 'Social support in the face of adversity: the role of cognitive appraisal.' *Journal of Research in Personality*, 23: 354–72.

34. Rotter, J. 1975. 'Some problems and misconceptions related to the construct of internal versus external control of reinforcements.' *Journal of Consulting and Clinical Psychology*, 43: 56–67.

35. Kobasa, S. C. 1979. 'Stressful life events, personality and health: an enquiry into hardiness.' *Journal of Personality and Social Psychology*, 37: 1–11.

36. Antonovsky, A. 1993. 'The structure and properties of the sense of coherence scale.' *Social Science and Medicine*, 36(6): 725–33.

37. Foa, E. B. & Rothbaum, B. O. 1998. *Treating the trauma of rape: cognitive behavioral therapy for PTSD*. New York: Guilford.

38. Brewin et al., 2000.

39. Kaufman, J., Yang, B., Douglas-Palumberi, H., Grasso, D., Lipschitz, D, Houshyar, S. et al. 2006. 'Brain-derived neurotrophic factor-5-HHTLPR gene interactions and environmental modifiers of depression in children.' *Biological Psychiatry*, 59(8): 673–80.

40. Herman, 1992.

41. Young, A. 1995. *The harmony of illusions: inventing posttraumatic stress disorder*. New Jersey: Princeton University Press.

42. Summerfield, D. 1995. 'Addressing human response to war and atrocity: major challenges in research and practices and the limitations of Western psychiatric models.' In R. J. Kleber, C. R. Figley & B. P. Gersons (eds). *Beyond trauma: cultural and societal dynamics*, pp. 17–30. New York: Plenum.
     Summerfield, D. 1999. 'A critique of seven assumptions behind psychological trauma programmes in war-affected areas.' *Social Science and Medicine*, 48(10): 1449–62.
     Summerfield, D. 2001. 'The invention of post-traumatic stress disorder and the usefulness of a psychiatric category.' *British Medical Journal*, 322(7278): 95–8.

43. Summerfield, 1995.

44. Summerfield, 2001, quote on page 95.

45. Eagle, G. (2002). 'The political conundrums of post-traumatic stress disorder.' In D. Hook & G. Eagle (eds.). *Psychopathology and social prejudice*, pp. 75–91. Cape Town: University of Cape Town Press.
     Kleinman, A. & Kleinman, J. 1996. 'The appeal of experience, the dismay of images: cultural appropriations of suffering in our times.' *Daedalus*, 125(1): xi–xx.
     Martin-Baró, I. 1994. *Writings for a liberation psychology*. Cambridge, MA: Harvard University Press.
     Summerfield, 2001.

46. Stein, D. J., Seedat, S., Iversen, A. & Wessely, S. 2007. 'Post-traumatic stress disorder: medicine and politics.' *Lancet*, 369(9556): 139–44.

47. Kessler et al., 1995.

48. Kessler et al., 1995.

49. Mayou R. & Bryant, B. 2001. 'Outcome in consecutive emergency department attenders following a road traffic accident.' *British Journal of Psychiatry*, 179: 528–34.
     Schnyder U., Moergeli H., Klaghofer R. & Buddeberg C. 2001. 'Incidence and prediction of posttraumatic stress disorder symptoms in severely injured accident victims.' *American Journal of Psychiatry*, 158: 594–9.

50. American Psychiatric Association, 2000.

51. Ibid.

52. Ouimette, P. & Brown, P. J. 2003. *Trauma and substance abuse: causes, consequences and treatment of comorbid disorders*. Washington, DC: American Psychological Association.

53. American Psychiatric Association, 2000.

54. Kessler et al., 1995.

55. Pelcovitz, D., van der Kolk, B., Roth, S., Mandel, F., Kaplan, S. & Resick, P. 1997. 'Development of a criteria set and a Structured Interview for Disorders of Extreme Stress (SIDES).' *Journal of Traumatic Stress*, 10(1): 3–16.
     Roth, S. H., Newman, E., Pelcovitz, D., van der Kolk, B. A. & Mandel, F. S. 1997. 'Complex PTSD in victims exposed to sexual and physical abuse:

results from the DSM-IV Field Trial for Posttraumatic Stress Disorder.' *Journal of Traumatic Stress*, 10(4): 539–55.

Van der Kolk, B. A. 1996*b*. 'The complexity of adaptation to trauma.' In B. A. van der Kolk, A. C. McFarlane & L. Weisaeth (eds). *Traumatic stress: the effects of overwhelming experience on mind, body and society*.(pp. 182–213). New York: Guilford Press.

56. Herman, 1992.

57. American Psychiatric Association, 2000.

58. World Health Organisation. 1992. *The ICD-10 classification of mental and behavioural disorders: clinical descriptions and diagnostic guidelines*. Geneva: WHO.

59. American Psychiatric Association, 2000.

60. Herman, 1992.

61. Roelofs, K. & Spinhoven, P. 2007. 'Trauma and medically unexplained symptoms: towards an integration of cognitive and neuro-biological accounts.' *Clinical Psychology Review*, 27: 798–820.

62. Wyatt, G. E., Guthrie, D. & Notgrass, C. M. 1992. 'Differential effects of women's child sexual abuse and subsequent sexual revictimisation.' *Journal of Consulting and Clinical Psychology*, 60(2): 167–73.

63. Ford, J. D. 2009. 'Neurobiological and developmental research: clinical implications.' In C. A. Courtois & J. D. Ford (eds). *Treating complex traumatic stress disorders: an evidence-based guide*. pp. 31–58. New York: Guilford Press.

64. Herman, 1992.
    Ford, 2009.

65. Straker, G. & the Sanctuaries Counselling Team, 1987. 'The continuous traumatic stress syndrome: the single therapeutic interview.' *Psychology in Society*, 8: 48–78.

66. Nicholas, L. J. 1990. 'The response of South African professional psychology associations to apartheid.' *Journal of the History of the Behavioral Sciences*, 26(1): 58–63.

67. Straker et al., 1987.

68. Foster, D., Davis, D. & Sandler, D. 1987. *Detention and torture in South Africa*. London: James Currey.

69. Michelson, C. 1994. 'Township violence, levels of distress, and post-traumatic stress disorder, among displacees from Natal.' *Psychology in Society*, 18: 47–59.

70. Bouwer, C. & Stein, D. 1998. 'Survivors of torture presenting at an anxiety disorders clinic: symptomatology and pharmacotherapy.' *Journal of Nervous and Mental Disease*, 186(5): 316–8.

71. Pillay, B. J. 2000. 'Providing mental health services to survivors: a KwaZulu-Natal perspective.' *Ethnicity and Health*, 5(3-4): 269–72.

72. Kaminer, D., Stein, D., Mbanga, I. & Zungu-Dirwayi, N. 2001. 'The Truth and Reconciliation Commission in South Africa: relation to psychiatric status and forgiveness among survivors of human rights violations.' *British Journal of Psychiatry*, 178: 373–7.

73. Zungu-Dirwayi, N., Kaminer, D., Mbanga, I. & Stein, D. J. 2004. 'The psychiatric sequelae of human rights violations: a challenge for primary health care.' *Journal of Nervous and Mental Disease*, 192(4): 255–9.

74. Kagee, A. 2004. 'Present concerns of survivors of human rights violations in South Africa.' *Social Science and Medicine*, 59(3): 625–35.

75. Gear, S. 2002. *Wishing us away: challenges facing ex-combatants in the 'new' South Africa*. Violence and Transition Series, 8. Johannesburg: Centre for the Study of Violence and Reconciliation.

76. Kaminer et al., 2008

77. Peltzer, K. 2000. 'Trauma symptom correlates of criminal victimization in an urban community sample, South Africa.' *Journal of Psychology in Africa, South of the Sahara, the Caribbean, and Afro-Latin-America*, 10(1): 49–62.

78. McGregor, J., Schoeman, W. J. & Stuart, A. D. 2002. 'The victim's experience of hijacking: an exploratory study.' *Health SA Gesondheid*, 7: 33–45.

79. Kaminer et al., 2008.

80. Marais, A., De Villiers, P. J. T., Möller, A. T. & Stein, D. J. 1999. 'Domestic violence in patients visiting general practitioners: prevalence, phenomenology, and association with psychopathology.' *South African Medical Journal*, 89: 635–40.

81. Mgoqi. N. C. 2006. 'The role of assault severity, sex role beliefs, personality factors, attribution style and psychological impact in predicting coping with rape victimization.' Unpublished doctoral dissertation. University of the Witwatersrand, Johannesburg.

82. Kaminer et al., 2008.

83. Welz, T., Hosegood, V., Jaffar, S., Batzing-Feigenbaum, J., Herbst, K. & Newell, M. 2007. 'Continued very high prevalence of HIV infection in rural KwaZulu-Natal, South Africa: a population-based longitudinal study.' *AIDS*, 21(11): 1467–72.

84. Leserman, J., Jackson, E. D., Pettito, J. M., Golden, R. N., Silva, S. G., Perkins, D. O. et al. 1995. 'Progression to AIDS: the effects of stress, depressive symptoms, and social support.' *Psychosomatic Medicine*, 61(3): 397–406.

85. Sternhell, P. S. & Corr, M. J. 2002. 'Psychiatric morbidity and adherence to antiretroviral medication in patiemts with HIV/AIDS.' *Australian and New Zealand Journal of Psychiatry*, 36(4): 528–33.

86. Olley, B., Seedat. S. & Stein, D. J. 2006. 'Persistence of psychiatric disorders in a cohort of HIV/AIDS patients in South Africa: a 6-month follow-up study.' *Journal of Psychosomatic Research*, 61(4): 479–84.

87. Myer, L., Smit, J., Le Roux, L., Parker, S, Stein, D. J. & Seedat, S. 2008. 'Common mental disorders among HIV-infected individuals in South Africa: prevalence, predictors and validation of brief psychiatric rating scales.' *AIDS Patient Care and STDs*, 22(2): 147–58.

88. Martin, L. & Kagee, A. 2008. 'Lifetime and HIV-related PTSD amongst persons recently diagnosed with HIV.' *AIDS and Behavior*, (consulted on 12 December 2008).

89. Peltzer, K. & Renner, W. 2004. 'Psychosocial correlates of the impact of road traffic accidents among South African drivers and passengers.' *Accident Analysis and Prevention*, 36: 367–74.

90. Seedat, S., le Roux, C. & Stein, D. J. 2004. 'Prevalence and characteristics of trauma and post-traumatic stress symptoms in operational members of the South Africa National Defence Force.' *Military Medicine*, 168: 71–75.

91. Jones, R. & Kagee, A. 2005. 'Predictors of post-traumatic stress symptoms among South African police personnel.' *South African Journal of Psychology*, 35: 209–24.
    Kopel, H. & Friedman, M. 1997. 'Post-traumatic stress symptoms in South African police exposed to violence.' *Journal of Traumatic Stress*, 10(2): 307–17.
    Peltzer, K. 2001. 'Stress and traumatic symptoms among police officers at a South African police station.' *Acta Criminologica*, 16: 21–6.

92. Carey, P. D., Stein. D. J., Zungu-Dirwayi, N. & Seedat, S. 2003. 'Trauma and posttraumatic stress disorder in an urban Xhosa primary care population: prevalence, comorbidity, and service use patterns.' *Journal of Nervous and Mental Disease*, 191(4): 230–6.

93. Peltzer, K., Seakamela, M. J., Manganye, L., Mamiane, K. G., Motsei, M. S. & Mathebula, T. T. M. 2007. 'Trauma and posttraumatic stress disorder in a rural primary care population in South Africa.' *Psychological Reports*, 100(3): 1115–20.

94. Kessler, R. C. & Ustun, T. B. 2004. 'The World Mental Health (WMH) Survey Initiative Version of the World Health Organization (WHO) Composite International Diagnostic Interview (CIDI).' *International Journal of Methods in Psychiatric Research*, 13(2): 93–121.

95. Stein et al., 2008.

96. Kessler et al., 1995.
    Breslau et al., 1998.

97. Norris et al., 2003.

98. Williams, S. L., Williams, D. R., Stein, D. J., Seedat, S., Jackson, P. B. & Moomal, H. 2007. 'Multiple traumatic events and psychological distress: The South Africa Stress and Health Study.' *Journal of Traumatic Stress*, 20(5): 845–55.

99. Griffin, M. G., Uhlmansiek, M. H., Resick, P. A. & Mechanic, M. B. 2004. 'Comparison of the post-traumatic stress disorder scale versus the clinician-administered post-traumatic stress disorder scale in domestic violence survivors.' *Journal of Traumatic Stress*, 17(6): 497–503.

100. Maw, A. 2009. 'Challenges in the selection of psychometric tools for the assessment of PTSD: a micro-study of data drawn from a longitudinal study on the psychological impact of rape trauma in the Western Cape.' Paper presented at Assessment and Management of the Mental Health Consequences of Trauma in South Africa: A Research Perspective, Cape Town, June.

101. Peltzer, K. 1998. 'Ethnocultural construction of posttraumatic stress symptoms in African contexts.' *Journal of Psychology in Africa, South of the Sahara, the Caribbean, and Afro-Latin-America*, 1: 17–30.

Chapter 4

1. Horowitz, M. S. 1992. *Stress response syndromes.* Northvale, N. J.: Jason Aronson.

2. Janoff-Bulman, J. 1992. *Shattered assumptions: towards a new psychology of trauma.* Toronto: Free Press.

3. Ibid.

4. Foa, E. B. & Rothbaum, B. O. 1998. *Treating the trauma of rape: cognitive behavioral therapy for PTSD.* New York: Guilford.

5. Ehlers, A. & Clark, D. M. 2000. 'A cognitive model of posttraumatic stress disorder.' *Behavior Research and Therapy*, 38(4): 319–45., Herman, J. L. 1992. *Trauma and recovery: from domestic abuse to political terror.* London: Pandora., Janoff-Bulman, 1992.

6. Tedeschi, R. G., Calhoun, L. G. & McCann, A. 2007. 'Evaluating resource gain: understanding and misunderstanding posttraumatic growth.' *Applied Psychology: An International Review*, 56(3): 396–406.

7. Janoff-Bulman, 1992.

8. Gergen, K. J. & Gergen, M. M. 1988. 'Narrative and the self as relationship.' In L. Berkowitz (ed.). *Advances in experimental social psychology, Vol. 1. Social psychological studies of the self: perspectives and programs*, pp. 17–56. San Diego, CA: Academic Press.
   Wigren, J. 1994. 'Narrative completion in the treatment of trauma.' *Psychotherapy*, 31(3): 415–23.

9. Bruner, J. S. 1990. *Acts of meaning.* Cambridge, MA.: Harvard University Press.

10. Janoff-Bulman, 1992.

11. Thacker, M. 2008. 'Meaning-making amongst South African survivors of violent crime.' Paper presented at the 14th South African Psychology Congress, Johannesburg, August.

12. Ehlers & Clark, 2000.
13. Everly, G. S. & Lating, J. M. 2004. *Personality-guided therapy for post traumatic stress disorder.* Washington: American Psychological Association. Wilson, J.P. & Moran, T.A. 1998. 'Psychological trauma: post traumatic stress disorder and spirituality.' *Journal of Psychology and Theology,* 26(2): 168–78.
14. Wilson & Moran, 1998.
15. Ogden, C. J., Kaminer, D., van Kradenburg, J., Seedat, S. & Stein, D. J. 2000. 'Narrative themes in responses to trauma in a religious community.' *Central African Journal of Medicine,* 46(7): 178–83.
16. Lipshitz, M. 2007. 'Meaning-making processes among bereaved mothers who have lost a child to cancer.' Unpublished Masters dissertation. University of Cape Town, Cape Town.
17. Everly & Lating, 2004.
    Herman, 1992.
18. Davidson, J., Connor, K. M. & Lee, L. 2005. 'Beliefs in karma and reincarnation among survivors of violent trauma: a community survey.' *Social Psychiatry and Psychiatric Epidemiology,* 40(2): 120–5.
19. Idemudia, E. S. 2009. 'Cultural dynamics of trauma expression and psychotherapy: the African perspective.' In S. N. Madu (ed.). *Trauma and psychotherapy in Africa,* pp. 43–50. Polokwane: University of Limpopo Press.
20. Eagle, G. 2005*a.* 'Therapy at the cultural interface: implications of African cosmology for traumatic stress intervention.' *Journal of Contemporary Psychotherapy,* 35(2): 199–210.
    Straker, G. 1994. 'Integrating African and Western healing practices in South Africa.' *American Journal of Psychotherapy,* 48(3): 455–67.
21. Eagle, 2005*a.*
22. Janoff-Bulman, 1992.
23. Silver, R. L., Boon, C. & Stones, M. 1983. 'Searching for meaning in misfortune: making sense of incest.' *Journal of Social Issues,* 39(2): 81–102.
24. Booley, A. 2008. 'Subjective accounts of post-rape adjustment amongst South African rape survivors.' Paper presented at the 14th South African Psychology Congress, Johannesburg, August.
25. Magwaza, A.S. 1999. 'Assumptive world of traumatised South African adults.' *Journal of Social Psychology,* 139(5): 622–30, quote on page 627.
26. Gobodo-Madikizela, P. 2002. 'Remorse, forgiveness, and rehumanization: stories from South Africa.' *Journal of Humanistic Psychology,* 42(1): 7–32.
    Truth and Reconciliation Commission, 1998. *Truth and Reconciliation Commission of South Africa Report, Vol. 5.* Cape Town: CTP.
27. Thacker, 2008.
28. Ehlers & Clark, 2000.

49. Tedeschi & Calhoun, 2004.
50. Ibid.
51. Ibid.
52. Polatinsky, S. & Esprey, Y. 2000. 'An assessment of gender differences in the perception of benefit finding resulting from the loss of a child.' *Journal of Traumatic Stress*, 13(4): 709–18.
53. Kaminer, D., Booley, A., Lipshitz, M. & Thacker, M. 2009. 'Post-trauma meaning making among South African survivors of different forms of trauma.' Paper presented at the Coping and Resilience International Conference, Dubrovnik/Cavtat, October.
54. Roe-Berning, S. 2009. 'The complexity of posttraumatic growth: evidence from a South African sample.' Unpublished Masters dissertation. University of the Witwatersrand, Johannesburg.
55. Linley, P.A. 2003. 'Positive adaptation to trauma: wisdom as both process and outcome.' *Journal of Traumatic Stress*, 16(6): 601–10.
56. Tedeschi & Calhoun, 2004.
57. Harvey, M. R., Mischler, E. G., Koenen, K. & Harney, P. A. 2000. 'In the aftermath of sexual abuse: making and remaking meaning in narratives of trauma and recovery.' *Narrative Inquiry*, 10(2): 291–311.
     Janoff-Bulman, R. & McPherson Frantz, C. 1997. 'The impact of trauma on meaning: from meaningless world to meaningful life.' In M. Power & R. Brewin (eds), *The transformation of meaning in psychological therapies: integrating theory and practice*, pp. 91–106. Chichester: Wiley.
     Tedeschi & Calhoun, 2004.
58. Lantz, J. & Lantz, J. 2001. 'Trauma therapy: a meaning centered approach.' *International Forum for Logotherapy*, 24(2): 68–76.
59. Linley, P. A. & Joseph, S. 2004. 'Positive change following trauma and adversity: a review.' *Journal of Traumatic Stress*, 17(1): 11–21.
     Helgeson, V. S., Reynolds, K. A. & Tomich, P. L. 2006. 'A meta-analytic review of benefit finding and growth.' *Special Issue: Benefit-Finding*, 74(5): 797–816.
     Zoellner, T. & Maercker, A. 2006. 'Posttraumatic growth in clinical psychology: a critical review and introduction of a two-component model.' *Clinical Psychology Review*, 26(5): 626–53.
60. Linley & Joseph, 2004.
     Helgeson et al., 2006.
     Zoellner & Maercker, 2006.
61. Tedeschi & Calhoun, 2004.
62. Ibid.
63. Butler, 2007.

64. Levine, S., Laufer, A., Hamama-Raz, Y., Stein, E. & Solomon, Z. 2008. 'Posttraumatic growth in adolescence: examining its components and relationship with PTSD.' *Journal of Traumatic Stress*, 21(5): 492–96.,
Powell, S., Rosner, R., Butollo, W., Tedeschi, R.G. & Calhoun L.G. 2003. 'Posttraumatic growth after war: a study with former refugees and displaced people in Sarajevo.' *Journal of Clinical Psychology*, 59: 71–83.
65. Zoellner & Maercker, 2006.

Chapter 5

1. Herman, J. L. 1992. *Trauma and recovery: from domestic abuse to political terror.* London: Pandora.
2. Friedman, M. 2004. *Post-traumatic stress disorder: the latest assessment and treatment strategies.* Kansas City: Compact Clinicals.
3. Raphael, B. & Dobson, M. 2001. 'Acute posttraumatic interventions.' In J. Wilson, M. Friedman & J. Lindy (eds.). *Treating psychological trauma and PTSD.* pp. 139–158. New York: The Guilford Press.
4. Ibid., quote on page 141.
5. Ibid., quote on page 145.
6. Mitchell, J. T. 1983. 'When disaster strikes.' *Journal of Emergency Medical Services*, 8: 36–9.
7. Dyregov, A. 1989. 'Caring for helpers in disaster situations: psychological debriefing.' *Disaster Management*, 2: 25–30.
8. Friedman, 2004.
9. Mitchell, J. T., 1983.
10. Horowitz, M. S. 1992. *Stress response syndromes.* Northvale, N. J.: Jason Aronson.
11. Dyregov, A. 1997. The process in psychological debriefings. *Journal of Traumatic Stress*, 10(4): 589–607.
12. Rose, S. & Bisson, J. 1998. 'Brief early psychological interventions following trauma: a systematic review of the literature.' *Journal of Traumatic Stress*, 11(4): 697–710, quote on page 698.
13. Ibid.
14. Ibid.
15. Foa, E., Rothbaum, B., Riggs, D. & Murdock, T. 1991. 'Treatment of posttraumatic stress disorder in rape victims: a comparison between cognitive-behavioural procedures and counselling.' *Journal of Consulting and Clinical Psychology*, 59(5): 715–23.
Foa, E. & Rothbaum, B. 1998. *Treating the trauma of rape.* New York: Guilford Press.
16. Resick, P. & Schnicke, M. 1992. 'Cognitive processing therapy for sexual assault victims.' *Journal of Consulting and Clinical Psychology*, 60(5): 748–56.

17. Meichenbaum, D. 1994. *A clinical handbook/practical therapist manual for assessing and treating adults with post-traumatic stress disorder (PTSD).* Waterloo, Ontario: Institute Press.
18. Ehlers, A. Clark, D., Hackmann, A., McManus, F. & Fennel, M. 2005. 'Cognitive therapy for post-traumatic stress disorder: development and evaluation.' *Behaviour Research and Therapy*, 43: 413–31.
19. Foa & Rothbaum, 1998.
20. Resick & Schnicke, 1992.
21. Meichenbaum, 1994.
22. Ehlers, A. & Clark, D. M. 2000. 'A cognitive model of post-traumatic stress disorder.' *Behaviour Research and Therapy*, 38: 319–45.
23. Rothbaum, B., Meadows, E., Resick, P. & Foy, D. W. 2000. 'Cognitive-behavioral therapy.' In E. B. Foa, T. M. Keane & M. J. Friedman (eds). *Effective treatments for PTSD: practice guidelines from the International Society for Traumatic Stress Studies*, pp. 60–83. New York: Guilford Press.
24. Draucker, C. B. 1998. 'Narrative therapy for women who have lived with violence.' *Archives of Psychiatric Nursing*, 12(3): 162–8.
    White, M. & Epston, D 1990. *Narrative means to therapeutic ends.* New York: W. W. Norton.
25. Merscham, C. 2000. 'Restorying trauma with narrative therapy: using the phantom family.' *Family Journal*, 8(3): 282–7, quote on page 284.
26. Neuner, F., Schauer, M., Klaschik, C., Karunakara, U. & Elbert, T. 2004. 'A comparison of narrative exposure therapy, supportive counselling and psychoeducation for treating posttraumatic stress disorder in an African refugee settlement.' *Journal of Consulting and Clinical Psychology*, 72(4): 579–87.
27. Meichenbaum, D. 1997. *Treating post-traumatic stress disorder: a handbook and practical manual for therapy.* Chichester: Wiley.
28. Agger, I. & Jensen, S. B. 1990. 'Testimony as ritual and evidence in psychotherapy for political refugees.' *Journal of Traumatic Stress*, 3(1): 115–130.
    Cienfuegos, A. J. & Monelli, C. 1983. 'The testimony of political repression as a therapeutic instrument.' *American Journal of Orthopsychiatry*, 53(1): 43–51.
29. Luebben, S. 2003. 'Testimony work with Bosnian refugees living in legal limbo.' *British Journal of Counselling and Development*, 31(4): 393–402.
    Igreja, V., Kleijn, W. C., Schreuder, B. J. N., van Dijk, J. A. & Verschuur, M. 2004. 'Testimony method to ameliorate post-traumatic stress symptoms: community-based intervention study with Mozambican civil war survivors.' *British Journal of Psychiatry*, 184: 251–7.

Weine, S. M., Kulenovic, A. D., Pavkovic, I. & Gibbons, R. 1998. 'Testimony psychotherapy in Bosnian refugees: a pilot study.' *American Journal of Psychiatry*, 155(12): 1720–6.

30. Kagee, A. 2006. 'The relationship between statement giving at the South African Truth and Reconciliation Commission and psychological distress among former political detainees.' *South African Journal of Psychology*, 36(1): 10–24.

Kaminer, D., Stein, D., Mbanga, I. and Zungu-Dirwayi, N. 2001. 'The Truth and Reconciliation Commission in South Africa: relation to psychiatric status and forgiveness among survivors of human rights violations.' *British Journal of Psychiatry*, 178: 373–7.

31. Krupnick, J. L. 1980. 'Brief psychotherapy for victims of violent crime.' *Victimology*, 5: 347–54.

32. Horowitz, 1992.

33. Lindy, J. 1996. 'Psychoanalytic psychotherapy of posttraumatic stress disorder.' In B. van der Kolk, A. MacFarlane & O. Weisaeth (eds). *Traumatic stress: the effects of overwhelming experience on mind, body and society*, pp. 525–36. New York: Guilford Press.

34. Peterson, P., Prout, M & Schwarz, R. 1991. *Posttraumatic stress disorder: a clinician's guide*. New York: Plenum Press.

35. Ibid., quote on page 136.

36. Friedman, 2004, quote on page 53.

37. Peterson et al, 1991, quote on page 156.

38. Krupnick, 1980.

39. Brom, D., Kleber, R. & Defares, P. 1989. 'Brief psychotherapy for post-traumatic stress disorder.' *Journal of Consulting and Clinical Psychology*, 57: 607–12.

40. Horowitz, 1992.

41. Meichenbaum, 1994.

42. Meichenbaum. 1994., cited in Edwards, D. (2005a). 'Treating PTSD in South African contexts: a theoretical framework and a model for developing evidence-based practice.' *Journal of Psychology in Africa*, 15(2): 209–220, quote on page 213.

43. Eagle, G. 2000. 'The shattering of the stimulus barrier: the case for an integrative approach in short-term treatment of psychological trauma.' *Journal of Psychotherapy Integration*, 10 (3): 301–24.

44 . Edwards, D. 2009. 'Treating posttraumatic stress disorder in South Africa: An integrative model grounded in case-based theory.' *Journal of Psychology in Africa*, 19 (2): 189–98, quote on page 190.

45. Eagle, 2000.

46. Prout, M. & Schwarz, R. 1991. 'Posttraumatic stress disorder: a brief integrated approach.' *International Journal of Short Term Psychotherapy*, 39: 113–24.
47. Cited in Eagle, 2000, quote on page 303.
48. Cited in Huber, C. 1997. 'PTSD – A search for active ingredients.' *Family Journal*, 5(2): 144–8.
49. Shapiro, F. 1989. 'Efficacy of eye movement and desensitisation procedure in the treatment of traumatic memories. *Journal of Traumatic Stress*, 2(2): 199–223.
     Shapiro, F. 1995. *Eye movement desensitisation and reprocessing: basic principles, protocols and procedures.* New York: Guilford Press.
50. Chemtob, C. M., Tolin, D. F., Van der Kolk, B. A. & Pitman, R. K. 2000. 'Eye movement desensitization and reprocessing.' In E. B. Foa, T. M. Keane & M. J. Friedman (eds). *Effective treatments for PTSD*, pp. 139–54. New York: Guilford Press.
51. Garland, C. (ed.). 1998. *Understanding trauma: a psychoanalytical approach.* London: Duckworth.
52. Horowitz, 1992.
53. Watts, J. & Eagle, G. 2002. 'When objects attack in reality: psychoanalytic contributions to formulations of the impact and treatment of traumatic stress incidences: Part II.' *Psychoanalytic Psychotherapy in South Africa*, 11: 8–13.
54. Garland, C. 1998. 'Thinking about trauma.' In C. Garland (ed.). *Understanding trauma: a psychoanalytical approach*, pp. 9–31. London: Karnac.
55. McCann, L. & Pearlman, L. 1990. *Trauma and the adult survivor.* New York: Brunner Mazel.
56. See Medical Foundation website, http//: www.torturecare.org.uk
57. See IRCT website, http/:www.irct.org
58. Grootenhuis, K. 2007. 'Therapeutic dilemmas in working with African refugees in South Africa.' Unpublished Masters dissertation. University of the Witwatersrand, Johannesburg.
59. See CSVR website, http//:www.csvr.org.za, for the full report.
60. Foa, Davidson & Frances, 1999, cited in Marotta, S. 2000. 'Best practices for counsellors who treat posttraumatic stress disorder.' *Journal of Counselling and Development*, 78(4): 492–6.
61. Southwick, S. & Yehuda, R. 1993. 'The interaction between pharmacotherapy and psychotherapy in the treatment of posttraumatic stress disorder.' *American Journal of Psychotherapy*, 47(3): 404–11.
62. Ibid., quote on page 408.
63. Marotta, 2000, quote on page 494.
64. Tucker, P. & Trautman, R. 2000. 'Understanding and treating PTSD: past, present and future.' *Bulletin of the Menninger Clinic*, 64(3): 37–52, quote on page 44.

65. Southwick & Yehuda, 1993.
66. Friedman, 2004.
67. Akinsulure-Smith, A. M. 2009. 'Brief psychoeducational group work treatment with re-traumatized refugees and asylum seekers.' *Journal for Specialists in Group Work*, 34 (2): 137–50.
68. Ibid., quote on page 58.
69. Friedman, 2004.
70. See National Peace Accord Trust website, http//:www.NPAT.org.za
71. Soderlund, J. 1999. 'Go wild: wilderness therapy for trauma.' *New Therapist*, 4: 32–3, quote on page 33.
72. See National Peace Accord Trust website.
73. *Themba Lesizwe* was an organisation set up with funding from the European Union aimed at establishing a National Network of Trauma Care Providers in South Africa and with hopes of creating wider Southern African links. The original partners were the CSVR Trauma Clinic, the Natal Survivors of Violence Project and the Cape Town Trauma Centre for Survivors of Torture and Violence. However, the organisation expanded to include other urban and rural bodies providing services of various kinds to trauma victims. *Themba Lesizwe* held several conferences to discuss trauma intervention programmes and initiatives and created a forum in which ideas could be shared. There was an effort to document best practice and to establish a common research data base of clients and interventions. Unfortunately the organisation could not be sustained after the funding ran out in 2006–07.
74. Khulumani, meaning 'speak out together', was the name of an organisation formed to give expression to victims of apartheid who had testified at the TRC or who had suffered from political violence but chose not to become involved with the TRC. It was a self-help group that played both a supportive and a lobbying function. For example, Kulumani arranged for memorial and remembrance services and held regular meetings at which members would share thoughts and feelings about their losses. In addition, Khulumani lobbied the government for reparation for victims of apartheid, and the organisation is still involved in a legal battle with large multinationals over apartheid exploitation and the need for reparation. The group worked initially under the auspices of the CSVR but then became an independent organisation and expanded from a Johannesburg base into other regions. The organisation has been less visible of late and seems to have lost some of its post-TRC momentum.
75. Friedman, 2004.
76. Tucker & Trautman, 2000, quote on page 43.
77. Marotta, 2000, quote on page 494.
78. Ibid.

79 . Cited in Tucker & Trautman, 2000, quote on page 44.

80. Tucker & Trautman, 2000.

81. Eagle, G. 2005*b*. 'Grasping the thorn: the impact and supervision of traumatic stress therapy in the South African context.' *Journal of Psychology in Africa*, 15(2): 197–208.

Edwards, D. 2005*a*.

Edwards, D. 2005*b*. 'Critical perspectives on research on post-traumatic stress disorder and implications for the South African context.' *Journal of Psychology in Africa*, 15(2):117–24.

82. Grootenhuis, 2007.

83. Straker, G. & the Sanctuaries Counselling Team. 1987. 'The continuous traumatic stress syndrome: the single therapeutic interview.' *Psychology in Society*, 8: 46–79.

84. Ibid.

85. Edwards, 2005*a*.

Straker, 1987.

86. Grootenhuis, 2007.

87. Eagle, G. 2005*a*. 'Therapy at the cultural interface: implications of African cosmology for traumatic stress intervention.' *Journal of Contemporary Psychotherapy*, 35(2): 199–210.

Straker, G. 1994. 'Integrating African and Western healing practices in South Africa.' *American Journal of Psychotherapy*, 48(3): 455–67.

88. Eagle, 2005*a*.

89. Louw, D. & Pretorius, E. 1995. 'The traditional healer in a multicultural society: The South African Experience.' In L. Adler & B. Mukerji (eds). *Spirit versus scalpel: Traditional healing and modern psychotherapy*, pp.41–57. Westport, Connecticut: Bergin & Garvey.

90. Benn, M. 2007. 'Perceived alterations in racial perceptions of victims of violent crime.' Unpublished Masters dissertation. University of the Witwatersrand, Johannesburg.

91. Ibid.

92. Sibisi, H. 2008. 'The understanding and approach of trained volunteer counsellors to negative racial sentiments in traumatized clients.' Unpublished Masters dissertation. University of the Witwatersrand, Johannesburg.

Fletcher, T. 2008. 'How do psychodynamically oriented therapists understand, respond to, and work with negative racial sentiments amongst traumatized clients?' Unpublished Masters dissertation. University of the Witwatersrand, Johannesburg.

93. Sibisi, 2008.

94. Fletcher, 2008.

95. Meintjes, B. 1999. 'Where violence has been: rural trauma work.' *New Therapist*, 4: 18–22.

96. Edwards, 2005*b*

97. Christie, K. 2000. *The South African Truth Commission*. Great Britain: Macmillan.
   Gibson, J. L. 2004. *Overcoming apartheid: can truth reconcile a divided nation?* Cape Town: HSRC Press.
   Stein, D., Seedat, S., Kaminer , D., Moomal, H., Herman, A., Sonnega, J. et al. 1998. 'Impact of the Truth and Reconciliation Commission on psychological distress and forgiveness in South Africa.' *Social Psychiatry and Psychiatric Epidemiology*, 43: 462–8.

98. Eagle, 2005*b*.
   Wilson, J. P. & Lindy, J. D. 1999. 'Empathic strain and countertransference. In M. J. Horowitz (ed.). *Essential papers on posttraumatic stress disorder*, pp. 518–43. New York: New York University Press.

99. Edwards, 2005*a*.

Chapter 6

1. Herman, J. L. 1992. *Trauma and recovery: from domestic abuse to political terror*. London: Pandora.

2. Myer, L., Stein, D., Jackson, P., Herman, A., Seedat, S. & Williams, D. 2009. 'Impact of common mental disorders during childhood and adolescence on secondary school completion.' *South African Medical Journal*, 99(5): 254–356.

3. Seedat, S., Nyamai, C., Njenga, F., Vythilingum, B. & Stein, D. 2004. 'Trauma exposure and post-traumatic stress symptoms in urban African schools: survey in Cape Town and Nairobi.' *British Journal of Psychiatry*, 184: 169–75.

4. Ensink, K., Roberstson, B., Zissis, C. & Leger, P. 1997. 'Post-traumatic stress disorder in children exposed to violence.' *South African Medical Journal*, 87(11): 1526–30.

5. Shields, N., Nadasen, K. & Pierce, L. 2008. 'The effects of community violence on children in Cape Town, South Africa.' *Child Abuse and Neglect*, 32: 589–601.

6. Ward, C. L., Flisher, A. J., Zissis, C., Muller, M. & Lombard, C. 2001. 'Exposure to violence and its relationship to psychopathology in adolescents.' *Injury Prevention*, 7: 297–301.

7. Ward, C., Martin, E., Theron, C. & Distiller, B. 2007. 'Factors affecting resilience in children exposed to violence.' *South African Journal of Psychology*, 37(1): 165–87.

8. Peltzer, K. 1999. 'Posttraumatic stress symptoms in a population of rural children in South Africa.' *Psychological Reports*, 85: 646–50.
9. Berton, M. & Stabb, S. 1996. 'Exposure to violence and post-traumatic stress disorder in urban adolescents.' *Adolescence*, 31(122): 489–98.
10. Seedat et al., 2004.
11. Cairns, E. & Dawes, A. 1996. 'Children: ethnic and political violence – a commentary.' *Child Development*, 67: 129–39.
12. Qouta, S., Punamaki, R. & El Sarraj, E. 2003. 'Prevalence and determinants of PTSD among Palestinian children exposed to military violence.' *European Journal of Child and Adolescent Psychiatry*, 12(6): 265–72.
13. Shannon, M., Lonigan, C., Finch, A. & Taylor, C. 1994. 'Children exposed to disaster: I. Epidemiology of post-traumatic symptoms and symptom profile.' *Journal of American Academy of Child and Adolescent Psychiatry*, 33(1): 80–93.
14. Bryant, R., Salmon, K., Sinclair, E. & Davidson, P. 2007. 'The relationship between acute stress disorder and posttraumatic stress disorder in injured children.' *Journal of Traumatic Stress*, 20(6): 1075–9.
15. American Psychiatric Association. 2000. *Diagnostic and statistical manual of mental disorders* (4th ed, text revision). Washington D.C.: American Psychiatric Association.
16. Dawes, A., Tredoux, C. & Feinstein, A. 1989. 'Political violence in South Africa: some effects on children of the violent destruction of their community.' *International Journal of Mental Health*, 18(2): 16–43.
    Magwaza, A. S., Killian, B. J., Petersen, I. & Pillay, Y. 1993. 'The effects of chronic violence on pre-school children living in South African townships.' *Child Abuse and Neglect*, 17: 795–803.
17. Straker, G. 1992. *Faces in the revolution: the psychological effects of violence on township youth in South Africa*. Cape Town: David Philip.
18. Ensink et al., 1997.
19. Seedat et al., 2004.
20. Carey, P., Walker, J., Rossouw, W., Seedat, S. & Stein, D. 2008. 'Risk indicators and psychopathology in traumatised children and adolescents with a history of sexual abuse.' *European Child and Adolescent Psychiatry*, 17(2): 93–98.
21. Peltzer, 1999.
22. Ward et al., 2001.
23. Barbarin, O. A., Richter, L. & deWet, T. 2001. 'Exposure to violence, coping resources and adjustment of South African children.' *American Journal of Orthopsychiatry*, 7: 16–25.
    Seedat et al., 2001.
    Ward et al., 2004.

24. Barbarin et al., 2001.

25. Cluver, L. & Gardner, F. 2006. 'The psychological well-being of children orphaned by AIDS in Cape Town, South Africa.' *Annals of General Psychiatry*, 5: 8–19, quote on page 8.

26. Duncan, N. & Rock, B. 1997*a*. 'Going beyond the statistics.' In B. Rock (ed.). *Spirals of suffering: public violence and children*, pp. 69–114. Pretoria: HSRC Publishers.

27. Emmet, T. 2003. 'Social disorganisation, social capital and violence prevention in South Africa.' *African Safety Promotion: A Journal of Injury and Violence Prevention*, 1(2): 4–18.

28. Qouta et al., 2003.
    Shannon et al., 1994.
    Yule, W. 2003. 'Early intervention strategies with traumatised children, adolescents and families.' In R. Orner and U. Schnyder (eds). *Reconstructing early interventions after trauma.* pp. 25–50. Oxford: Oxford University Press.

29. Nader, K. O. 1997. 'Assessing traumatic experiences in children.' In J. Wilson and T. Keane (eds). *Assessing psychological trauma and PTSD.* pp.291–348. New York: The Guilford Press.

30. Nader, 1997, quote on page 306.

31. Terr, L. 1991. 'Childhood trauma: an outline and overview.' *American Journal of Psychiatry*, 148(1): 10–20.

32. Ibid.

33. Ibid.

34. Ibid.

35. American Psychiatric Association, 2000.

36. Ibid.

37. Terr, 1991.

38. Ibid.

39. Ibid.

40. Eth, S. & Pynoos, R. S. 1985. 'Developmental perspectives on psychic trauma in childhood.' In C. Figley (ed.). *Trauma and its wake*, pp. 36–52. New York: Brunner Mazel.

41. Erikson, E. 1950. *Childhood and society*. New York: Norton.

42. Yule, W., Perrin, S. & Smith, P. 1999. 'Post-traumatic stress disorders in children and adolescents.' In W. Yule (ed.). *Post-traumatic stress disorders: concepts and therapy*, pp. 25–50. Chichester: John Wiley and Sons.

43. Reported in interview with school principal on 702 radio station in early March, 2008. The school march was also documented in local newspaper, *The Northcliff Melville Times*, 10–16 March, 2008.

44. American Academy of Child and Adolescent Psychiatry 1998. 'Practice parameters for the assessment and treatment of children and adolescents

with posttraumatic stress disorder.' *Journal of the American Academy of Child and Adolescent Psychiatry*, 37(Supp.): 4–26.

45. Barbarin et al., 2001.
    Dawes, A. & Tredoux, C. 1989. 'Emotional status of children exposed to political violence in the Crossroads squatter area during 1986/87.' *Psychology in Society*, 12: 33–47.
46. Qouta et al., 2003, quote on page 265.
47. Gil-Rivas, V., Chen Silver, R., Holman, E., McIntosh & Poulin, M. 2007. 'Parental response and adolescent adjustment to the September 11, 2001 terrorist attacks.' *Journal of Traumatic Stress*, 20(6): 1063–8.
48. Levy, S. & Lemma, A. 2004. 'The impact of trauma on the psyche: internal and external processes.' In S. Levy & A. Lemma (eds). *The perversion of loss – psychoanalytic perspectives on trauma*, pp. 50–70. New York: Brunner Routledge.
49. Janoff-Bulman, J. 1992. *Shattered assumptions: towards a new psychology of trauma*. Toronto: Free Press.
50. Rock, B. 1997. 'Introduction.' In B. Rock (ed.). *Spirals of suffering: public violence and children*, pp. i–v. Pretoria: HSRC Publishers, quote on page v.
51. Butchart, A., Phinney, A., Check, P. & Villaveces, A. 2004. *Preventing violence: a guide to implementing the recommendations of the World Report on Violence and Health. Report of the Department of Injuries and Violence prevention*. Geneva: World Health Organisation.
52. Duncan, N. & Rock, B. 1997*b*. 'Overview.' In B. Rock (ed.). *Spirals of suffering: public violence and children*, pp. 31–42. Pretoria: HSRC Publishers, quote on page 33.
53. B. Rock. 1997.
54. Duncan, N. & Rock, B. 1997*c*. 'Children and violence: quantifying the damage.' In B. Rock (ed.). *Spirals of suffering: public violence and children*, pp. 43–67. Pretoria: HSRC Publishers.
55. Langa, M. & Eagle, G. 2008. 'The intractability of militarised masculinity: a case study of former combatants in the Kathorus area, South Africa.' *South African Journal of Psychology*, 38(1): 152–75.
56. Cluver & Gardner, 2006.
57. Ibid., quote on page 13.
58. Ibid., quote on page 13.
59. Cluver, L., Fincham, D. & Seedat, S. 2009. 'Posttraumatic stress in Aids-orphaned children exposed to high levels of trauma: the protective role of perceived social support.' *Journal of Traumatic Stress*, 22(2): 106–112.
60. Yule, 2003.
61. Seedat, S., Stein, D., Ziervogel, C., Middleton, T., Kaminer, D., Emsley, R. & Rossouw, W. 2002. 'Comparison of response to a selective serotonin

reuptake inhibitor in children, adolescents, and adults with posttraumatic stress disorder.' *Journal of Child and Adolescent Psychopharmacology*, 12(1): 37–46.

62. Cohen, J. A., Berliner, L. & March, J. S. 2000*a*. 'Treatment of children and adolescents.' In E. B. Foa, T. M. Keane & M.J. Friedman (eds.). *Effective treatments for PTSD: practice guidelines from the International Society for Traumatic Stress Studies*, pp. 106–38. New York: Guilford.
   Cohen, J. A., Berliner, L. & March, J. S. 2000*b*. 'Treatment guidelines: Treatment of children and adolescents.' In E. B. Foa, T. M. Keane & M.J. Friedman (eds). *Effective treatments for PTSD: practice guidelines from the International Society for Traumatic Stress Studies*, pp. 330–2. New York: Guilford.

63. Pynoos, R. S. & Eth, S. 1986. 'Witness to violence: the child interview.' *Journal of the American Academy of Child and Adolescent Psychiatry*, 25(3): 306–19.

64. American Academy of Child and Adolescent Psychiatry, 1998.
   Cohen et al., 2000*b*.

65. Yule, 2003.

66. Leibowitz, S., Mendelsohn, M. & Michelson, C. 1999. 'Child rape: extending the therapeutic intervention to include the mother-child dyad.' *South African Journal of Psychology*, 29: 103–18.

67. See National Peace Accord Trust website, http/:www.NPAT.co.za

68. See REPSSI website, http//:www.REPSSI.co.za

69. Shields et al., 2008.

70. Ward et al., 2007.

71. The South African Institute for Journalism Studies has recently been looking into policy in this regard.

Chapter 7

1. See South African Human Rights Commission website for report, http//:www. sahrc.org.za

2. Manson, S. P. 1997. 'Cross-cultural and multiethnic assessment of trauma.' In J. P. Wilson & T. M. Keane (eds). *Assessing psychological trauma and PTSD*, pp. 239–66. London: Guilford Press.
   Marsella, A. J., Friedman, M. J. & Huland Spain, E. 1996. 'Ethnocultural aspects of PTSD: an overview of issues and research directions.' In A. J. Marsella, M. J. Friedman, E. T. Gerrity & R.M. Scurfield (eds). *Ethnocultural aspects of posttraumatic stress disorder: issues, research and clinical applications*, pp. 105–30. Washington, DC: American Psychological Association.
   Stamm, B. H. & Friedman, M. J. 2000. 'Cultural diversity in the appraisal

and expression of trauma.' In A. Y. Shalev, R. Yehuda & A. C. McFarlane (eds.). *International handbook of human response to trauma*, pp. 69–85. New York: Kluwer.

3. Kim, U. & Berry, J. W. 1993. 'Introduction.' In U. Kim & J. W. Berry (eds). *Indigenous psychologies: research experience in cultural context*, pp. 1–29. Newbury Park: Sage.
    Manson, 1997.

4. Kleinman, A. 1986. *Social origins of distress and disease*. New Haven: Yale University Press.
    Lewis-Fernandez, R. & Kleinman, A. 1995. 'Cultural psychiatry: theoretical, clinical and research issues.' *Psychiatric Clinics of North America*, 18(3): 433–48.
    Swartz, L. 1998. *Culture and mental health: a Southern African view*. Cape Town: Oxford University Press.

5. Peltzer, K. 1998. 'Ethnocultural construction of posttraumatic stress symptoms in African contexts.' *Journal of Psychology in Africa, South of the Sahara, the Caribbean, and Afro-Latin-America*, 1: 17–30.

6. De Jong, J. T. V. M., Komproe, I. H., Spinazzola, J., van der Kolk, B. & Van Ommeren, M. H. 2005. 'DESNOS in three postconflict settings: assessing cross-cultural construct equivalence.' *Journal of Traumatic Stress*, 18(1): 13–22.

7. Kaminer, D., Grimsrud, A., Myer, L., Stein, D. & Williams, D. R. 2008. 'Risk for posttraumatic stress disorder associated with different forms of interpersonal violence in South Africa.' *Social Science and Medicine*, 67: 1589–95.

8. Norman, R., Matzopoulos, R., Groenewald, P. & Bradshaw, D. 2007. 'The high burden of injuries in South Africa.' *Bulletin of the World Health Organisation*, 85(9): 649–732.

9. Swartz, 1998.

10. Kagee, A. 2004. 'Present concerns of survivors of human rights violations in South Africa.' *Social Science and Medicine*, 59(3): 625–35.

11. Farmer, P. 1996. 'On suffering and structural violence: a view from below.' *Daedalus*, 125(1): 261–83.
    Swartz, 1998.

BIBLIOGRAPHY

Abrahams, N., Jewkes, R., Laubscher, R. & Hoffman, M. 2006. 'Intimate partner violence: prevalence and risk factors for men in Cape Town, South Africa.' *Violence and Victims*, 21(2): 247–64.

Abrahams, N., Jewkes, R., Martin, L.J., Mathews, S., Vetten, L. & Lombard, C. 2009. 'Mortality of women from intimate partner violence in South Africa: a national epidemiological study.' *Violence and Victims*, 24(4): 546–56.

Abrahams, N., Martin, L. J., Jewkes, R., Mathews, S., Vetten, L. & Lombard, C. 2008. 'The epidemiology and the pathology of rape homicide in South Africa.' *Forensic Science International*, 178(2-3): 132–8.

Abrahams, N., Martin, L. J. & Vetten, L. 2004. 'An overview of gender-based violence in South Africa and South African responses.' In S. Suffla, A. van Niekerk & N. Duncan (eds). *Crime, violence and injury prevention in South Africa: developments and challenges*, pp. 40–64. Tygerberg: Medical Research Council-University of South Africa Crime, Violence and Injury Lead Programme.

Agger, I. & Jensen, S. B. 1990. 'Testimony as ritual and evidence in psychotherapy for political refugees.' *Journal of Traumatic Stress*, 3(1): 115–30.

Akinsulure-Smith, A. M. 2009. 'Brief psychoeducational group treatment with re-traumatized refugees and asylum seekers.' *Journal for Specialists in Group Work*, 34(2): 137–50.

Altbeker, A. 2007. *A country at war with itself: South Africa's crisis of crime.* Johannesburg: Jonathan Ball.

American Academy of Child and Adolescent Psychiatry. 1998. 'Practice parameters for the assessment and treatment of children and adolescents with posttraumatic stress disorder.' *Journal of the American Academy of Child and Adolescent Psychiatry*, 37 (Supp.): 4-26.

American Psychiatric Association. 2000. *Diagnostic and statistical manual of mental disorders* (4th ed., text revision). Washington DC: APA.

Amnesty International. 2007. *Annual Report 2007*. London: Amnesty International Publications.

Andrews, B., Brewin, C. R. & Rose, S. 2003. 'Gender, social support and PTSD in victims of violent crime.' *Journal of Traumatic Stress*, 16(4): 421–7.

Antonovsky, A. 1993. 'The structure and properties of the sense of coherence scale.' *Social Science and Medicine*, 36(6): 725–33.

Artz, L. 1999. *Violence against women in rural Southern Cape: exploring access to justice through a feminist jurisprudence framework*. Institute of Criminology, University of Cape Town, Cape Town, South Africa.

Barbarin, O. A., Richter, L. & deWet, T. 2001. 'Exposure to violence, coping resources and adjustment of South African children.' *American Journal of Orthopsychiatry*, 71(1): 16–25.

Benn, M. 2007. 'Perceived alterations in racial perceptions of victims of violent crime.' Unpublished Masters dissertation. University of the Witwatersrand, Johannesburg.

Bennett, K. K., Compas, B. E., Beckford, E. & Glinder, J. G. 2005. 'Self-blame and distress among women with newly diagnosed breast cancer.' *Journal of Behavioural Medicine*, 28(4): 313–23.

Berton, M. & Stabb, S. 1996. 'Exposure to violence and post-traumatic stress disorder in urban adolescents.' *Adolescence*, 31 (122): 489–98.

Bollen, S., Artz, L., Vetten, L. & Louw, A. 1999. *Violence against women in metropolitan South Africa: a study on impact on service delivery* (Monograph No. 41). Johannesburg: Institute for Security Studies.

Bonanno, G. A., Galea, S. Bucciarelli, A. & Vlahov, D. 2007. 'What predicts psychological resilience after disaster? The role of demographics, resources and life stress.' *Journal of Consulting and Clinical Psychology*, 75(5): 671–82.

Booley, A. 2008. 'Subjective accounts of post-rape adjustment amongst South African rape survivors.' Paper presented at the 14th South African Psychology Congress, Johannesburg, August.

Bouwer, C., & Stein, D. 1998. 'Survivors of torture presenting at an anxiety disorders clinic: Symptomatology and pharmacotherapy.' *Journal of Nervous and Mental Disease*, 186(5): 316–8.

Bradshaw, D., Groenewald, P., Laubscher, R., Nannan, N., Nojilana, B. & Norman, R. 2003. *Initial burden of disease estimates for South Africa, 2000*. Tygerberg: Medical Research Council.

Breslau, N. 1998. 'Epidemiology of trauma and posttraumatic stress disorder.' In R. Yehuda (ed.). *Review of psychiatry, Vol. 17*, pp. 1–30. Washington, DC: American Psychiatric Association.

Breslau, N. 2002. 'Epidemiologic studies of trauma, posttraumatic stress disorder and other psychiatric disorders.' *Canadian Journal of Psychiatry*, 47(10): 923–9.

Breslau, N., Kessler, R. C., Chilcoat H. D., Schultz, L. R., Davis, G. C. & Andreski, P. 1998. 'Trauma and posttraumatic stress disorder in the community: The 1996 Detroit Area Survey of Trauma.' *Archives of General Psychiatry*, 55(7): 626–32.

Brewin, C. R., Andrews, B. & Valentine, J. D. 2000. 'Meta-analysis of risk factors for posttraumatic stress disorder in trauma-exposed adults.' *Journal of Consulting and Clinical Psychology*, 68(5): 748–66.

Brewin, C. R., MacCarthy, B. & Furnham, A. 1989. 'Social support in the face of adversity: the role of cognitive appraisal.' *Journal of Research in Personality*, 23(3): 354–72.

Brom, D., Kleber, R. & Defares, P. 1989. 'Brief psychotherapy for posttraumatic stress disorder.' *Journal of Consulting and Clinical Psychology*, 57(5): 607–12.

Bruner, J. S. 1990. *Acts of meaning.* Cambridge, MA.: Harvard University Press.

Bryant, R., Salmon, K., Sinclair, E. & Davidson, P. 2007. 'The relationship between acute stress disorder and posttraumatic stress disorder in injured children.' *Journal of Traumatic Stress*, 20 (6): 1075–9.

Buga, G. A. B., Amoko, D. H. A. & Ncayiyana, D. 1996. 'Sexual behaviour, contraceptive practices and reproductive health among school adolescents in rural Transkei.' *South African Medical Journal*, 86(5): 523–7.

Burrows, S., Bowman, B., Matzopoulus, R. & van Niekerk, A. 2001. *A profile of fatal injuries in South Africa 2000. Second Annual Report of the National Injury Mortality Surveillance System.* Tygerberg: Medical Research Council.

Burton, P. 2006. 'Easy prey: results of the national youth victimisation study.' *SA Crime Quarterly*, 16(June): 1–6.

Butchart, A., Phinney, A., Check, P. & Villaveces, A. 2004. *Preventing violence: a guide to implementing the recommendations of the World Report on Violence and Health. Report of the Department of Injuries and Violence prevention.* Geneva: World Health Organisation.

Butler, L. D. 2007. 'Growing pains: commentary on the field of posttraumatic growth and Hobfoll and colleagues' recent contribution to it.' *Applied Psychology: An International Review*, 56(13): 367–78.

Cairns, E. & Dawes, A. 1996. 'Children: ethnic and political violence – a commentary.' *Child Development*, 67(1): 129–39.

Carey, P. D., Stein. D. J., Zungu-Dirwayi, N. & Seedat, S. 2003. 'Trauma and posttraumatic stress disorder in an urban Xhosa primary care population: prevalence, comorbidity, and service use patterns.' *Journal of Nervous and Mental Disease*, 191(4): 230–6.

Carey, P., Walker, J., Rossouw, W., Seedat, S. & Stein, D. 2008. 'Risk indicators and psychopathology in traumatised children and adolescents with a history of sexual abuse.' *European Child and Adolescent Psychiatry*, 17(2): 93–8.

Chemtob, C. M., Tolin, D. F., van der Kolk, B. A. & Pitman, R. K. 2000. 'Eye movement desensitization and reprocessing.' In E. B. Foa, T. M. Keane &

M. J. Friedman (eds). *Effective treatments for PTSD.* pp. 139–54. New York: Guilford Press.

Christie, K. 2000. *The South African Truth Commission.* Great Britain: Macmillan.

Cienfuegos, A. J. & Monelli, C. 1983. 'The testimony of political repression as a therapeutic instrument.' *American Journal of Orthopsychiatry*, 53(1): 43–51.

Cluver, L., Fincham, D. & Seedat, S. 2009. 'Posttraumatic stress in Aids-orphaned children exposed to high levels of trauma: The protective role of perceived social support.' *Journal of Traumatic Stress*, 22(2): 106–12.

Cluver, L. & Gardner, F. 2006. 'The psychological well-being of children orphaned by AIDS in Cape Town, South Africa.' *Annals of General Psychiatry*, 5(8): 8–19.

Cohen, J. A., Berliner, L. & March, J. S. 2000*a*. 'Treatment of children and adolescents'. In E. B. Foa, T. M. Keane & M.J. Friedman (eds). *Effective treatments for PTSD: practice guidelines from the International Society for Traumatic Stress Studies*, pp. 106–38. New York: Guilford.

Cohen, J. A., Berliner, L. & March, J. S. 2000*b*. 'Treatment guidelines: treatment of children and adolescents.' In E. B. Foa, T. M. Keane & M.J. Friedman (eds). *Effective treatments for PTSD: Practice guidelines from the International Society for Traumatic Stress Studies*, pp. 330–2. New York: Guilford.

Coleman, M. 1998. *A crime against humanity: analysing the repression of the apartheid state.* Johannesburg: Human Rights Commission.

Collings, S. J. 1995. 'The long-term effects of contact and non-contact forms of child sexual abuse in a sample of university men.' *Child Abuse and Neglect*, 19(1): 1–6.

Collings, S. J. 1997. 'Child sexual abuse in a sample of South African women students: prevalence, characteristics and long-term effects.' *South African Journal of Psychology*, 27(1): 37–42.

Collings, S. J. 2005. 'Sexual abuse of boys in KwaZulu-Natal South Africa: a hospital-based study.' *Journal of Child and Adolescent Mental Health*, 17(1): 23–5.

Creamer, M., Burgess, P. & McFarlane, A.C. 2001. 'Post-traumatic stress disorder: findings from the Australian National Survey of Mental Health and Well-being.' *Psychological Medicine*, 31(7): 1237–47.

Davidson, J., Connor, K. M. and Lee, L. 2005. 'Beliefs in karma and reincarnation among survivors of violent trauma: a community survey.' *Social Psychiatry and Psychiatric Epidemiology*, 40(2): 120–5.

Dawes, A., Long, W., Alexander, L. & Ward, C. L. 2006. *A situation analysis of children affected by maltreatment and violence in the Western Cape. A case report for the Research Directorate, Department of Social Services and Poverty Alleviation: Provincial Government of the Western Cape.* Cape Town: Human Sciences Research Council.

Dawes, A. & Tredoux, C. 1989. 'Emotional status of children exposed to political violence in the Crossroads squatter area during 1986/87.' *Psychology in Society*, 12: 33–47.

Dawes, A., Tredoux, C. & Feinstein, A. 1989. 'Political violence in South Africa: some effects on children of the violent destruction of their community.' *International Journal of Mental Health*, 18(2): 16–43.

De Jong, J. T. V. M., Komproe, I. H., Spinazzola, J., van der Kolk, B. & Van Ommeren, M. H. 2005. 'DESNOS in three postconflict settings: assessing cross-cultural construct equivalence.' *Journal of Traumatic Stress*, 18(1): 13–22.

Department of Health. 2002. *South Africa Demographic and Health Survey 1998: final report*. Pretoria: Department of Health.

Draucker, C. B. 1998. 'Narrative therapy for women who have lived with violence.' *Archives of Psychiatric Nursing*, 12(3): 162–8.

Duncan, N. & Rock, B. 1997a. 'Going beyond the statistics.' In B. Rock (ed.). *Spirals of suffering: public violence and children*, pp. 69–114. Pretoria: HSRC Publishers.

Duncan, N. & Rock, B. 1997b. 'Overview.' In B. Rock (ed.). *Spirals of suffering: public violence and children*, pp. 31–42. Pretoria: HSRC Publishers.

Duncan, N. & Rock, B. 1997c. 'Children and violence: quantifying the damage.' In B. Rock (ed.). *Spirals of suffering: public violence and children*, pp. 43–67. Pretoria: HSRC Publishers.

Dunkle, K. L., Jewkes, R. K., Brown, H. C., Gray, G. E., McIntyre, J. A. & Harlow, S. D. 2004. 'Gender-based violence, relationship power, and risk of HIV infection in women attending antenatal clinics in South Africa.' *Lancet*, 363(9419): 1415–21.

Dunkle, K. L., Jewkes, R. K., Nduna, M., Levin, J., Jama, N., Khuzwayo, N., Koss, M. P. & Duvvury, N. 2006. 'Perpetration of partner violence and HIV risk behaviour among young men in the rural Eastern Cape, South Africa.' *AIDS*, 20(16): 2107–14.

Dyregov, A. 1989. 'Caring for helpers in disaster situations: psychological debriefing.' *Disaster Management*, 2(1): 25–30.

Dyregov, A. 1997. 'The process in psychological debriefings.' *Journal of Traumatic Stress*, 10 (4): 589–607.

Eagle, G. 2000. 'The shattering of the stimulus barrier: the case for an integrative approach in short-term treatment of psychological trauma.' *Journal of Psychotherapy Integration*, 10 (3): 301–324.

Eagle, G. 2002. 'The political conundrums of post-traumatic stress disorder.' In D. Hook & G. Eagle (eds). *Psychopathology and social prejudice*, pp. 75–91. Cape Town: University of Cape Town Press.

Eagle, G. 2005a. 'Therapy at the cultural interface: implications of African cosmology for traumatic stress intervention.' *Journal of Contemporary Psychotherapy*, 35(2): 199–210.

Eagle, G. 2005*b*. 'Grasping the thorn: the impact and supervision of traumatic stress therapy in the South African context.' *Journal of Psychology in Africa*, 15(2): 197–208.

Edwards, D. 2005*a*. 'Treating PTSD in South African contexts: a theoretical framework and a model for developing evidence-based practice.' *Journal of Psychology in Africa*, 15(2): 209–220.

Edwards, D. 2005*b*. 'Critical perspectives on research on post-traumatic stress disorder and implications for the South African context.' *Journal of Psychology in Africa*, 15(2):117–24.

Edwards, D. 2009. 'Treating posttraumatic stress disorder in South Africa: An integrative model grounded in case based research.' *Journal of Psychology in Africa*, 19(2): 189–98.

Ehlers, A. & Clark, D. M. 2000. 'A cognitive model of posttraumatic stress disorder.' *Behavior Research and Therapy*, 38(4): 319–45.

Ehlers, A., Clark, D., Hackmann, A., McManus, F. & Fennel, M. 2005. 'Cognitive therapy for post-traumatic stress disorder: development and evaluation.' *Behaviour Research and Therapy*, 43(4): 413–31.

Emmet, T. 2003. 'Social disorganisation, social capital and violence prevention in South Africa.' *African Safety Promotion: A Journal of Injury and Violence Prevention*, 1(2): 4–18.

Ensink, K., Roberstson, B., Zissis, C. & Leger, P. 1997. 'Post-traumatic stress disorder in children exposed to violence.' *South African Medical Journal*, 87(11): 1526–30.

Erikson, E. 1950. *Childhood and society*. New York: Norton.

Esprey, Y. 1996. 'Post-traumatic stress and dimensions of trauma.' Unpublished Masters dissertation. University of the Witwatersrand, Johannesburg.

Eth, S. & Pynoos, R. S. 1985. 'Developmental perspectives on psychic trauma in childhood.' In C. Figley (ed.). *Trauma and its wake, Vol. 1*, pp. 36–52. New York: Brunner Mazel.

Everly, G. S. & Lating, J. M. 2004. *Personality-guided therapy for poststraumatic stress disorder*. Washington: American Psychological Association.

Farmer, P. 1996. 'On suffering and structural violence: a view from below.' *Daedalus*, 125(1): 261–83.

Finkelhor, D. 1994. 'Current information on the scope and nature of child sexual abuse.' *The Future of Children*, 4(2): 31–53.

Finkelhor, D. & Jones, L. 2006. 'Why have child maltreatment and child victimization declined?' *Journal of Social Issues*, 62(4): 685–716.

Fletcher, T. 2008. 'How do psychodynamically oriented therapists understand, respond to, and work with negative racial sentiments amongst traumatized clients?' Unpublished Masters dissertation. University of the Witwatersrand, Johannesburg.

Foa, E. B. & Rothbaum, B. O. 1998. *Treating the trauma of rape: cognitive behavioral therapy for PTSD*. New York: Guilford.

Foa, E., Rothbaum, B., Riggs, D. & Murdock, T. 1991. 'Treatment of posttraumatic stress disorder in rape victims: a comparison between cognitive-behavioural procedures and counselling.' *Journal of Consulting and Clinical Psychology*, 59(5): 715–23.

Ford, J. D. 2009 'Neurobiological and developmental research: clinical implications.' In C. A. Courtois & J. D. Ford (eds). *Treating complex traumatic stress disorders: an evidence-based guide*, pp. 31–58. New York: Guilford Press.

Foster, D., Davis, D., & Sandler, D. 1987. *Detention and torture in South Africa*. London: James Currey.

Frankl, V. 1964. *Man's search for meaning: an introduction to logotherapy*. New York: Simon and Schuster.

Frazier, P. A. 2000. 'The role of attributions and perceived control in recovery from rape.' *Journal of Personal and Interpersonal Loss*, 5(2-3): 203–25.

Frenkl, L. 2008. 'A support group for parents of burned children: a South African children's hospital burns unit.' *Burns*, 34(4): 565–9.

Freud, S. 1920/1948. *Beyond the pleasure principle*. London: Hogarth Press.

Friedman, M. J. 2003. *Post-traumatic stress disorder: the latest assessment and treatment strategies*. Kansas City: Compact Clinicals.

Garland, C. (ed.). 1998. *Understanding trauma: a psychoanalytical approach*. London: Duckworth.

Garland, C. 1998. 'Thinking about trauma.' In C. Garland (ed.). *Understanding trauma: a psychoanalytical approach*, pp. 9–31. London: Karnac.

Gear, S. 2002. *Wishing us away: challenges facing ex-combatants in the 'new' South Africa*. Violence and Transition Series, 8. Johannesburg: Centre for the Study of Violence and Reconciliation.

Gergen, K. J. & Gergen, M. M. 1988. 'Narrative and the self as relationship.' In L. Berkowitz (ed.). *Advances in experimental social psychology, Vol. 1: social psychological studies of the self: perspectives and programs*, pp. 17–56. San Diego, CA: Academic Press.

Gibson, J. L. 2004. *Overcoming apartheid: can truth reconcile a divided nation?*. Cape Town: HSRC Press.

Gil-Rivas, V., Chen Silver, R., Holman, E., McIntosh & Poulin, M. 2007. 'Parental response and adolescent adjustment to the September 11, 2001 terrorist attacks. *Journal of Traumatic Stress*, 20(6): 1063–8.

Gobodo-Madikizela, P. 2002. 'Remorse, forgiveness, and rehumanization: stories from South Africa.' *Journal of Humanistic Psychology*, 42(1): 7–32.

Griffin, M. G., Uhlmansiek, M. H., Resick, P. A. & Mechanic, M. B. 2004. 'Comparison of the post-traumatic stress disorder scale versus the clinician-administered post-traumatic stress disorder scale in domestic violence survivors.' *Journal of Traumatic Stress*, 17(6): 497–503.

Grootenhuis, K. 2007. 'Therapeutic dilemmas in working with African refugees in South Africa.' Unpublished Masters dissertation. University of the Witwatersrand, Johannesburg.

Guay, S., Billette, V. & Marchand, A. 2006. 'Exploring the links between posttraumatic stress disorder and social support: processes and potential research avenues.' *Journal of Traumatic Stress*, 19(3): 327–38.

Gupta, J., Silverman, J. G., Hemenway, D., Acevedo-Garcia, D., Stein, D. J. & Williams, D. R. 2008. 'Physical violence against intimate partners and related exposures to violence among South African men.' *CMAJ*, 179(6): 535–41.

Harvey, M. R., Mischler, E. G., Koenen, K. & Harney, P. A. 2000. 'In the aftermath of sexual abuse: making and remaking meaning in narratives of trauma and recovery.' *Narrative Inquiry*, 10(2): 291–311.

Heaven, P. C. L., Connors, J. & Pretorius, A. 1998. 'Victim characteristics and attribution of rape blame in Australia and South Africa.' *Journal of Social Psychology*, 138(1): 131–3.

Heise, L., Ellsberg, M. & Gottemoeller, M. 1999. *Ending violence against women*. Baltimore: The John Hopkins University School of Public Health.

Helgeson, V. S., Reynolds, K. A. & Tomich, P. L. 2006. 'A meta-analytic review of benefit finding and growth.' *Special Issue: Benefit-Finding*, 74(5): 797–816.

Herman, J. 1992. *Trauma and recovery: from domestic abuse to political terror*. London: Pandora.

Horowitz, M. S. 1992. *Stress response syndromes*. Northvale, N. J.: Jason Aronson.

Huber, C. 1997. 'PTSD: a search for active ingredients.' *Family Journal*, 5(2): 144–8.

Human Rights Watch. 1995. *Violence against women in South Africa: state response to domestic violence and rape*. New York/Washington: Human Rights Watch.

Idemudia, E. S. 2009. 'Cultural dynamics of trauma expression and psychotherapy: the African perspective.' In S. N. Madu (ed.). *Trauma and psychotherapy in Africa*, pp. 43–50. Polokwane: University of Limpopo Press.

Igreja, V., Kleijn, W. C., Schreuder, B. J. N., van Dijk, J. A. & Verschuur, M. 2004. 'Testimony method to ameliorate post-traumatic stress symptoms: community-based intervention study with Mozambican civil war survivors.' *British Journal of Psychiatry*, 184(3): 251–7.

Janet, P. 1919/1925. *Psychological healing, Vol 1*. Trans. E. Paul and C. Paul. New York: Macmillan.

Janoff-Bulman, J. 1992. *Shattered assumptions: towards a new psychology of trauma*. Toronto: Free Press.

Janoff-Bulman, R., & McPherson Frantz, C. 1997. 'The impact of trauma on meaning: from meaningless world to meaningful life.' In M. Power & R. Brewin (eds). *The transformation of meaning in psychological therapies: integrating theory and practice*, pp. 91–106. Chichester: Wiley.

Jewkes, R. & Abrahams, N. 2002. 'The epidemiology of rape and sexual coercion in South Africa: an overview.' *Social Science and Medicine*, 55(7): 1231–44.

Jewkes, R., Levin, J., Mbananga, N. & Bradshaw, D. 2002. 'Rape of girls in South Africa.' *Lancet*, 359(9303): 319–20.

Jewkes, R., Penn-Kekana, L., Levin, J., Ratsaka, M. & Schreiber, M. 2001. 'Prevalence of emotional, physical and sexual abuse of women in three South African provinces.' *South African Medical Journal*, 91(5): 421–8.

Jewkes, R., Sikweyiya, Y., Morrell, R. & Dunkle, K. 2009. *Understanding men's health and use of violence: interface of rape and HIV in South Africa.* Tygerberg: Medical Research Council Gender and Health Research Unit.

Jones, R. & Kagee, A. 2005. 'Predictors of post-traumatic stress symptoms among South African police personnel.' *South African Journal of Psychology*, 35(2): 209–24.

Kagee, A. 2004. 'Present concerns of survivors of human rights violations in South Africa.' *Social Science and Medicine*, 59(3): 625–35.

Kagee, A. 2006. 'The relationship between statement giving at the South African Truth and Reconciliation Commission and psychological distress among former political detainees.' *South African Journal of Psychology*, 36(1): 10–24.

Kaminer, D., Booley, A., Lipshitz, M. & Thacker, M. 2009. 'Post-trauma meaning making among South African survivors of different forms of trauma.' Paper presented at the Coping and Resilience International Conference, Dubrovnik/Cavtat, October.

Kaminer, D., Grimsrud, A., Myer, L., Stein, D. & Williams, D. R. 2008. 'Risk for posttraumatic stress disorder associated with different forms of interpersonal violence in South Africa.' *Social Science and Medicine*, 67(10): 1589–95.

Kaminer, D. & Seedat, S. 2005. 'Posttraumatic stress disorder.' In S. Romans & M. V. Seeman (eds.). *Women's mental health: a life-cycle approach*, pp. 221–36. Baltimore: Lippincott, Williams and Wilkins.

Kaminer, D., Stein, D., Mbanga, I. & Zungu-Dirwayi, N. 2001. 'The Truth and Reconciliation Commission in South Africa: relation to psychiatric status and forgiveness among survivors of human rights violations.' *British Journal of Psychiatry*, 178(4): 373–7.

Kaufman, J., Yang, B., Douglas-Palumberi, H., Grasso, D., Lipschitz, D, Houshyar, S., Krystal, J. H. & Gelernter, J. 2006. 'Brain-derived neurotrophic factor-5-HHTLPR gene interactions and environmental modifiers of depression in children.' *Biological Psychiatry*, 59(8): 673–80.

Kessler, R. C., Sonnega, A., Bromet, E., Hughes, M., & Nelson, C. B. 1995. 'Posttraumatic stress disorder in the National Comorbidity Survey.' *Archives of General Psychiatry*, 52(12): 1048–60.

Kessler, R. C. & Ustun, T. B. 2004. 'The World Mental Health (WMH) Survey Initiative Version of the World Health Organization (WHO) Composite International Diagnostic Interview (CIDI).' *International Journal of Methods in Psychiatric Research*, 13(2): 93–121.

Kilpatrick, D. G., Resnick, H. S., Freedy, J. R., Pelcovitz, D., Resick, P. A. & Roth, S. 1998. 'The posttraumatic stress disorder field trial: evaluation of the PTSD construct - criteria A through E.' In T. Widiger, A. Frances, H. Pincus, R. Ross, M. B. First & W. W. Davis (ed.). *DSM-IV sourcebook, Vol. 4*, pp. 803–44. Washington, DC: American Psychiatric Association Press.

Kim, U. & Berry, J. W. 1993. 'Introduction.' In U. Kim & J. W. Berry (eds). *Indigenous psychologies: research experience in cultural context*, pp. 1–29. Newbury Park: Sage.

Kimerling, R. & Calhoun, K. S. 1994. 'Somatic symptoms, social support, and treatment seeking among sexual assault victims.' *Journal of Consulting and Clinical Psychology*, 62(2): 333–40.

Kleinman, A. 1986. *Social origins of distress and disease*. New Haven: Yale University Press.

Kleinman, A. & Kleinman, J. 1996. 'The appeal of experience, the dismay of images: cultural appropriations of suffering in our times.' *Daedalus*, 125(1): xi–xx.

Kobasa, S. C. 1979. 'Stressful life events, personality and health: an enquiry into hardiness.' *Journal of Personality and Social Psychology*, 37(1): 1–11.

Kopel, H. & Friedman, M. 1997. 'Post-traumatic stress symptoms in South African police exposed to violence.' *Journal of Traumatic Stress*, 10(2): 307–17.

Krupnick, J. L. 1980. 'Brief psychotherapy for victims of violent crime.' *Victimology*, 5: 347–54.

Langa, M. & Eagle, G. 2008. 'The intractability of militarised masculinity: a case study of former combatants in the Kathorus area, South Africa.' *South African Journal of Psychology*, 38(1): 152–75.

Lantz, J. & Lantz, J. 2001. 'Trauma therapy: a meaning centered approach.' *International Forum for Logotherapy*, 24(2): 68–76.

Lebowitz, L. & Roth, S. 1994. '"I feel like a slut": the cultural context and women's response to being raped.' *Journal of Traumatic Stress*, 7(3): 363–90.

Leibowitz, S., Mendelsohn, M. & Michelson, C. 1999. 'Child rape: extending the therapeutic intervention to include the mother-child dyad.' *South African Journal of Psychology*, 29(3): 103–18.

Leserman, J., Jackson, E. D., Pettito, J. M., Golden, R. N., Silva, S. G., Perkins, D. O., Cai, J., Folds, J. D. & Evans, D. L. 1995. 'Progression to AIDS: the effects of stress, depressive symptoms, and social support.' *Psychosomatic Medicine*, 61(3): 397–406.

Levine, S., Laufer, A., Hamama-Raz, Y., Stein, E. & Solomon, Z. 2008. 'Posttraumatic growth in adolescence: examining its components and relationship with PTSD.' *Journal of Traumatic Stress*, 21(5): 492–6.

Levy, S. & Lemma, A. 2004. 'The impact of trauma on the psyche: internal and external processes.' In S. Levy & A. Lemma (eds.). *The perversion of loss – psychoanalytic perspectives on trauma*, pp. 50–70. New York: Brunner Routledge.

Lewis-Fernandez, R. & Kleinman, A. 1995. 'Cultural psychiatry: theoretical, clinical and research issues.' *Psychiatric Clinics of North America*, 18(3): 433–48.

Lindy, J. 1996. 'Psychoanalytic psychotherapy of posttraumatic stress disorder.' In B. van der Kolk, A. MacFarlane & O. Weisaeth (eds). *Traumatic stress: the effects of overwhelming experience on mind, body and society*, pp. 525–36. New York: Guilford Press.

Linley, P.A. 2003. 'Positive adaptation to trauma: wisdom as both process and outcome.' *Journal of Traumatic Stress*, 16(6): 601–10.

Linley, P. A. & Joseph, S. 2004. 'Positive change following trauma and adversity: a review.' *Journal of Traumatic Stress*, 17(1): 11–21.

Lipshitz, M. 2007. 'Meaning-making processes among bereaved mothers who have lost a child to cancer.' Unpublished Masters dissertation. University of Cape Town, Cape Town.

Louw, D. & Pretorius, E. 1995. 'The traditional healer in a multicultural society: The South African Experience.' In L. Adler & B. Mukerji (eds). *Spirit versus scalpel: Traditional healing and modern psychotherapy*, pp.41–57. Westport, Connecticut: Bergin & Garvey.

Ludsin, H. & Vetten, L. 2005. *Spiral of entrapment: abused women in conflict with the law*. Johannesburg: Jacana Media.

Luebben, S. 2003. 'Testimony work with Bosnian refugees living in legal limbo.' *British Journal of Counselling and Development*, 31(4): 393–402.

MacNair, R. M. 2002. 'Perpetration-induced traumatic stress in combat veterans.' *Peace and Conflict: Journal of Peace Psychology,* 8(1): 63–72.

Madu, S. N. 2001. 'The prevalence and patterns of childhood sexual abuse and victim-perpetrator relationship among a sample of university students.' *South African Journal of Psychology*, 31(4): 32–7.

Madu, S. N. & Peltzer, K. 2000. 'Risk factors and child sexual abuse among secondary school students in the Northern Province (South Africa).' *Child Abuse and Neglect*, 24(2): 259–68.

Magwaza, A. S. 1999. 'Assumptive world of traumatised South African adults.' *Journal of Social Psychology*, 139(5): 622–30.

Magwaza, A. S., Killian, B. J., Petersen, I. & Pillay, Y. 1993. 'The effects of chronic violence on pre-school children living in South African townships.' *Child Abuse and Neglect*, 17(6): 795–803.

Maiden, R. & Terreblanche-Lourens, P. 2006. 'Managing the trauma of community violence and workplace accidents in South Africa.' *Journal of Workplace Behavioral Health*, 21(3-4): 89–100.

Manson, S. P. 1997. 'Cross-cultural and multiethnic assessment of trauma.' In J. P. Wilson & T. M. Keane (eds.), *Assessing psychological trauma and PTSD*, pp. 239–66. London: Guilford Press.

Marais, A., De Villiers, P. J. T., Möller, A. T. & Stein, D. J. 1999. 'Domestic violence in patients visiting general practitioners: prevalence, phenomenology, and association with psychopathology.' *South African Medical Journal*, 89(6): 635–40.

Marotta, S. 2000. 'Best practices for counsellors who treat posttraumatic stress disorder.' *Journal of Counselling and Development*, 78(4): 492–6.

Marsella, A. J., Friedman, M. J. & Huland Spain, E. 1996. 'Ethnocultural aspects of PTSD: an overview of issues and research directions.' In A. J. Marsella, M. J. Friedman, E. T. Gerrity & R. M. Scurfield (eds.). *Ethnocultural aspects of posttraumatic stress disorder: issues, research and clinical applications*, pp. 105–30. Washington, DC: American Psychological Association.

Martin, L. 1999. 'Violence against women: an analysis of the epidemiology and patterns of injury in rape homicide in Cape Town and in rape in Johannesburg.' Unpublished Masters dissertation. University of Cape Town, Cape Town.

Martin, L. & Kagee, A. 2008. 'Lifetime and HIV-related PTSD amongst persons recently diagnosed with HIV.' *AIDS and Behavior*, (consulted on 12 December 2008 from http://www.springerlink.com/content/y5556882w5472722).

Martin-Baró, I. 1994. *Writings for a liberation psychology*. Cambridge, MA: Harvard University Press.

Masuku, S. 2002. 'Prevention is better than cure.' *SA Crime Quarterly*, 2(November): 1–7.

Matzopoulos, R., Norman, R. & Bradshaw, D. 2004. 'The burden of injury in South Africa: fatal injury trends and international comparisons.' In S. Suffla, A., van Niekerk & N. Duncan (eds). *Crime, violence and injury prevention in South Africa: developments and challenges*, pp. 9–21. Tygerberg: Medical Research Council-University of South Africa Crime, Violence and Injury Lead Programme.

Maw, A. 1990. 'Challenges in the selection of psychometric tools for the assessment of PTSD: a micro-study of data drawn from a longitudinal study on the psychological impact of rape trauma in the Western Cape.' Paper presented at Assessment and Management of the Mental Health Consequences of Trauma in South Africa: A Research Perspective. Cape Town, June.

Mayou R. & Bryant, B. 2001. 'Outcome in consecutive emergency department attenders following a road traffic accident.' *British Journal of Psychiatry*, 179(6): 528–34.

McCann, L. & Pearlman, L. 1990. *Trauma and the adult survivor*. New York: Brunner Mazel.

McFarlane, A. & van der Kolk, B. 1996. 'Trauma and its challenge to society.' In B. A. van der Kolk, A. C. McFarlane & L. Weisaeth (eds.). *Traumatic stress: the effects of overwhelming experience on mind, body and society*, pp. 24–46. New York: Guilford Press.

McGregor, J., Schoeman, W. J. & Stuart, A. D. 2002. 'The victim's experience of hijacking: an exploratory study.' *Health SA Gesondheid*, 7(1): 33–45.

Meichenbaum, D. 1994. *A clinical handbook/practical therapist manual for assessing and treating adults with post-traumatic stress disorder (PTSD).* Waterloo, Ontario: Institute Press.

Meichenbaum, D. 1997. *Treating post-traumatic stress disorder: a handbook and practical manual for therapy.* Chichester: Wiley.

Meintjes, B. 1999. 'Where violence has been: rural trauma work.' *New Therapist,* 4(1): 18–22.

Merscham, C. 2000. 'Restorying trauma with narrative therapy: using the phantom family.' *Family Journal of Counselling and Therapy for Children and Families,* 8(3): 282–7.

Mgoqi, N. C. 2006. 'The role of assault severity, sex role beliefs, personality factors, attribution style and psychological impact in predicting coping with rape victimization.' Unpublished Doctoral dissertation. University of the Witwatersrand, Johannesburg.

Michelson, C. 1994. 'Township violence, levels of distress, and post-traumatic stress disorder, among displacees from Natal.' *Psychology in Society,* 18(2): 47–59.

Mitchell, J. T. 1983. 'When disaster strikes.' *Journal of Emergency Medical Services,* 8(1): 36–9.

Myer, L., Smit, J., Le Roux, L., Parker, S, Stein, D. J. & Seedat, S. 2008. 'Common mental disorders among HIV-infected individuals in South Africa: prevalence, predictors and validation of brief psychiatric rating scales.' *AIDS Patient Care and STDs,* 22(2): 147–58.

Myer, L., Stein, D., Jackson, P., Herman, A., Seedat, S. & Williams, D. 2009. 'Impact of common mental disorders during childhood and adolescence on secondary school completion.' *South African Medical Journal,* 99(5): 354–6.

Nader, K. O. 1997. 'Assessing traumatic experiences in children.' In J. Wilson & T. Keane (eds). *Assessing psychological trauma and PTSD,* pp. 291–348. New York: The Guilford Press

Neuner, F., Schauer, M., Klaschik, C., Karunakara, U. & Elbert, T. 2004. 'A comparison of narrative exposure therapy, supportive counselling and psychoeducation for treating posttraumatic stress disorder in an African refugee settlement.' *Journal of Consulting and Clinical Psychology,* 72(4): 579–87.

Nicholas, L. J. 1990. 'The response of South African professional psychology associations to apartheid.' *Journal of the History of the Behavioral Sciences,* 26(1): 58–63.

Norman, R., Matzopoulos, R., Groenewald, P. & Bradshaw, D. 2007. 'The high burden of injuries in South Africa.' *Bulletin of the World Health Organization,* 85(9): 649–732.

Norris, F. H., Murphy, A. D. Baker, C. K., Perilla, J. L., Gutierrez Rodriguez, F. & Gutierrez Rodriguez, J. 2003. 'Epidemiology of trauma and posttraumatic stress disorder in Mexico.' *Journal of Abnormal Psychology,* 112(4): 646–56.

O'Brien, L.S. 1998. *Traumatic events and mental health.* Cambridge: University Press.

Ogden, C. J., Kaminer, D., van Kradenburg, J., Seedat, S. & Stein, D. J. 2000. 'Narrative themes in responses to trauma in a religious community.' *Central African Journal of Medicine,* 46(7): 178–83.

Olley, B., Seedat. S. & Stein, D. J. 2006. 'Persistence of psychiatric disorders in a cohort of HIV/AIDS patients in South Africa: a 6-month follow-up study.' *Journal of Psychosomatic Research,* 61(4): 479–84.

Ouimette, P. & Brown, P. J. 2003. *Trauma and substance abuse: causes, consequences and treatment of comorbid disorders.* Washington, D. C.: American Psychological Association.

Pelcovitz, D., van der Kolk, B., Roth, S., Mandel, F., Kaplan, S., & Resick, P. 1997. 'Development of a criteria set and a Structured Interview for Disorders of Extreme Stress (SIDES).' *Journal of Traumatic Stress,* 10(1): 3–16.

Peltzer, K. 1998. 'Ethnocultural construction of posttraumatic stress symptoms in African contexts.' *Journal of Psychology in Africa, South of the Sahara, the Caribbean, and Afro-Latin-America,* 1: 17–30.

Peltzer, K. 1999. 'Posttraumatic stress symptoms in a population of rural children in South Africa.' *Psychological Reports,* 85(2): 646–50.

Peltzer, K. 2000. 'Trauma symptom correlates of criminal victimization in an urban community sample, South Africa.' *Journal of Psychology in Africa, South of the Sahara, the Caribbean, and Afro-Latin-America,* 10(1): 49–62.

Peltzer, K. 2001. 'Stress and traumatic symptoms among police officers at a South African police station.' *Acta Criminologica,* 16(3): 21–6.

Peltzer, K. & Renner, W. 2004. 'Psychosocial correlates of the impact of road traffic accidents among South African drivers and passengers.' *Accident Analysis and Prevention,* 36(3), 367–74.

Peltzer, K., Seakamela, M. J., Manganye, L., Mamiane, K. G., Motsei, M. S. & Mathebula, T. T. M. 2007. 'Trauma and posttraumatic stress disorder in a rural primary care population in South Africa.' *Psychological Reports,* 100(3): 1115–20.

Peterson, P., Prout, M & Schwarz, R. 1991. *Posttraumatic stress disorder: a clinician's Guide.* New York: Plenum Press.

Piaget, J. 1962. *Play, dreams and imitation in childhood.* New York: Norton.

Piaget, J. & Inhelder, B. 1969. *The psychology of the child.* New York: Basic.

Pillay, B. J. 2000. 'Providing mental health services to survivors: a KwaZulu-Natal perspective.' *Ethnicity and Health,* 5(3-4): 269–72.

Pitman, R. K., Gilbertson, M. W., Gurvits, T. V., May, F. S., Lasko, N. B., Metzger, L. J., Shenton, M. E., Yehuda, R. & Orr, S.P. 2006. 'Clarifying the origin of biological abnormalities in PTSD through the study of identical twins discordant for combat exposure.' *Annals of the New York Academy of Sciences,* 1071: 242–54.

Polatinsky, S. & Esprey, Y. 2000. 'An assessment of gender differences in the perception of benefit finding resulting from the loss of a child.' *Journal of Traumatic Stress*, 13(4): 709–18.

Powell, S., Rosner, R., Butollo, W., Tedeschi, R. G. & Calhoun L. G. 2003. 'Posttraumatic growth after war: a study with former refugees and displaced people in Sarajevo.' *Journal of Clinical Psychology*, 59(1): 71–83.

Prout, M. & Schwarz, R. 1991. 'Posttraumatic stress disorder: a brief integrated approach.' *International Journal of Short Term Psychotherapy*, 39: 113–24.

Pynoos, R. S. & Eth, S. 1986. 'Witness to violence: the child interview.' *Journal of the American Academy of Child and Adolescent Psychiatry*, 25(3): 306–19.

Qouta, S, Punamaki, R. & El Sarraj, E. 2003. 'Prevalence and determinants of PTSD among Palestinian children exposed to military violence.' *European Journal of Child and Adolescent Psychiatry*, 12(6): 265–72.

Raphael, B. & Dobson, M. 2001. 'Acute posttraumatic interventions.' In J. Wilson, M. Friedman & J. Lindy (eds). *Treating psychological trauma and PTSD*, pp. 139–58. New York: The Guilford Press.

Ratele, K., Swart, L. & Seedat, M. 2009. 'Night-time fatal violence in South Africa.' In P. Hadfield (ed.). *Nightlife and crime: social order and governance in international perspective*, pp. 277–93. London: Oxford University Press.

Resick, P. A. 1993. 'The psychological impact of rape.' *Journal of Interpersonal Violence*, 8(2): 223–55.

Resick, P. & Schnicke, M. 1992. 'Cognitive processing therapy for sexual assault victims.' *Journal of Consulting and Clinical Psychology*, 60(5): 748–56.

Richter, L. 1996. *A survey of reproductive health issues among urban black youth in South Africa: final grant report*. Pretoria: Medical Research Council.

Rock, B. 1997. 'Introduction.' In B. Rock (ed.). *Spirals of suffering: public violence and children*, pp. i–v. Pretoria: HSRC Publishers.

Roe-Berning, S. 2009. *The complexity of posttraumatic growth: evidence from a South African sample.'* Unpublished Masters dissertation. University of the Witwatersrand, Johannesburg.

Roelofs, K. & Spinhoven, P. 2007. 'Trauma and medically unexplained symptoms: towards an integration of cognitive and neuro-biological accounts.' *Clinical Psychology Review*, 27(7): 798–820.

Rothbaum, B., Meadows, E., Resick, P. & Foy, D. W. 2000. 'Cognitive-behavioral therapy.' In E. B. Foa, T. M. Keane & M. J. Friedman (eds.). *Effective treatments for PTSD: practice guidelines from the International Society for Traumatic Stress Studies*, pp. 60–83. New York: Guilford Press.

Rose, S. & Bisson, J. 1998. 'Brief early psychological interventions following trauma: a systematic review of the literature.' *Journal of Traumatic Stress*, 11(4): 697–710.

Roth, S. H., Newman, E., Pelcovitz, D., van der Kolk, B. A. & Mandel, F. S. 1997. 'Complex PTSD in victims exposed to sexual and physical abuse: results from the DSM-IV Field Trial for Posttraumatic Stress Disorder.' *Journal of Traumatic Stress*, 10(4): 539–55.

Rotter, J. 1975. 'Some problems and misconceptions related to the construct of internal versus external control of reinforcements.' *Journal of Consulting and Clinical Psychology*, 43(1): 56–67.

Schnyder, U., Moergeli, H., Klaghofer, R. & Buddeberg C. 2001. 'Incidence and prediction of posttraumatic stress disorder symptoms in severely injured accident victims.' *American Journal of Psychiatry*,158: 594–9.

Seedat, M., Van Niekerk, A., Jewkes, R., Suffla, S. & Ratele, K. 2009. 'Violence and injuries in South Africa: prioritising an agenda for prevention.' *Lancet Special Issue: Health in South Africa*, 374(9694): 68–79.

Seedat, S., le Roux, C. & Stein, D. J. 2004. 'Prevalence and characteristics of trauma and post-traumatic stress symptoms in operational members of the South Africa National Defence Force.' *Military Medicine*, 168(1): 71–5.

Seedat, S., Nyamai, C., Njenga, F., Vythilingum, B. & Stein, D. 2004. 'Trauma exposure and post-traumatic stress symptoms in urban African schools: survey in Cape Town and Nairobi.' *British Journal of Psychiatry*, 184: 169–75.

Seedat, S., Stein, D., Ziervogel, C., Middleton, T., Kaminer, D., Emsley, R. & Rossouw, W. 2002. 'Comparison of response to a selective serotonin reuptake inhibitor in children, adolescents, and adults with posttraumatic stress disorder.' *Journal of Child and Adolescent Psychopharmacology*, 12(1): 37–46.

Seedat, S., van Noord, E., Vythilingum, B., Stein D. J. & Kaminer, D. 2000. 'School survey of exposure to violence and posttraumatic stress symptoms in adolescents.' *South African Journal of Child and Adolescent Mental Health*, 12(1): 38-44.

Shannon, M., Lonigan, C., Finch, A. & Taylor, C. 1994. 'Children exposed to disaster: I. Epidemiology of post-traumatic symptoms and symptom profiles.' *Journal of American Academy of Child and Adolescent Psychiatry*, 33(1): 80–93.

Shapiro, F. 1989. 'Efficacy of eye movement and desensitisation procedure in the treatment of traumatic memories.' *Journal of Traumatic Stress*, 2(2): 199–223.

Shapiro, F. 1995. *Eye movement desensitisation and reprocessing: basic principles, protocols and procedures*. New York: Guilford Press.

Shaw, M. 2002. *Crime and policing in post-apartheid South Africa: transformation under fire*. London: Hurst and Co.

Shields, N., Nadasen, K. & Pierce, L. 2008. 'The effects of community violence on children in Cape Town, South Africa.' *Child Abuse and Neglect*, 32(5): 589–601.

Sibisi, H. 2008. 'The understanding and approach of trained volunteer counsellors to negative racial sentiments in traumatized clients.' Unpublished Masters dissertation. University of the Witwatersrand, Johannesburg.

Silver, R. L., Boon, C., & Stones, M. 1983. 'Searching for meaning in misfortune: making sense of incest.' *Journal of Social Issues*, 39(2): 81–102.

Soderlund, J. 1999. 'Go wild: wilderness therapy for trauma.' *New Therapist*, 4: 32–33.

Southwick, S. & Yehuda, R. 1993. 'The interaction between pharmacotherapy and psychotherapy in the treatment of posttraumatic stress disorder.' *American Journal of Psychotherapy*, 47(3): 404–11.

Stamm, B. H. & Friedman, M. J. 2000. 'Cultural diversity in the appraisal and expression of trauma.' In A. Y. Shalev, R. Yehuda & A. C. McFarlane (ed.). *International handbook of human response to trauma*, pp. 69–85. New York: Kluwer.

Standing A. 2005. *The threats of gangs and anti-gangs policy: policy discussion paper.* Institute for Security Studies: Pretoria.

Stein, D., Cloitre, M., Nemeroff, C. B., Nutt, D. J., Seedat, S., Shalev, A., Wittchen, H.U. & Zohar, J. 2009. 'Cape Town consensus on posttraumatic stress disorder.' *CNS Spectrums*, 14(1): 52–8.

Stein, D., Seedat, S., Herman, A., Moomal, H., Heeringa, S. G., Kessler, R. C., Sonnega, J. & Williams, D.R. 2008. 'Lifetime prevalence of psychiatric disorders in South Africa.' *British Journal of Psychiatry*, 192(8): 112–7.

Stein, D. J., Seedat, S., Iversen, A. & Wessely, S. 2007. 'Post-traumatic stress disorder: medicine and politics.' *Lancet*, 369(9556): 139–44.

Stein, D., Seedat, S., Kaminer, D., Moomal, H., Herman, A., Sonnega, J., & Williams, D. R. 2008. 'Impact of the Truth and Reconciliation Commission on psychological distress and forgiveness in South Africa.' *Social Psychiatry and Psychiatric Epidemiology,* 43: 462–8.

Stein, D. J., Williams, S. L., Jackson, P. B. Seedat, S., Myer, L., Herman, A., Williams, D. R. 2009. 'Perpetration of gross human rights violations in South Africa: association with psychiatric disorders.' *South African Medical Journal*, 99(5 Pt 2): 390–5.

Stein, M., Walker, J., Hazen, A. & Forde, D. 1997. 'Full and partial posttraumatic stress disorder: findings from a community survey.' *American Journal of Psychiatry*, 154(8): 1114–9.

Steinberg, J. 2004. *The number.* Jonathan Ball: Johannesburg.

Sternhell, P. S. & Corr, M. J. 2002. 'Psychiatric morbidity and adherence to antiretroviral medication in patients with HIV/AIDS.' *Australian and New Zealand Journal of Psychiatry*, 36(4): 528–33.

Straker, G. 1992. *Faces in the revolution: the psychological effects of violence on township youth in South Africa.* Cape Town: David Philip.

Straker, G. 1994. 'Integrating African and Western healing practices in South Africa.' *American Journal of Psychotherapy*, 48(3): 455–67.

Straker, G. & The Sanctuaries Counselling Team. 1987. 'The continuous traumatic stress syndrome: the single therapeutic interview.' *Psychology in Society*, 8: 48–78.

Sukhai, A., Noah, M. & Prinsloo, M. 2004. 'Road traffic injury in South Africa: an epidemiological overview for 2001.' In S. Suffla, A. van Niekerk & N. Duncan (eds). *Crime, violence and injury prevention in South Africa: developments and challenges*, pp. 114–27. Tygerberg: Medical Research Council-University of South Africa Crime, Violence and Injury Lead Programme.

Summerfield, D. 1995. 'Addressing human response to war and atrocity: major challenges in research and practices and the limitations of Western psychiatric models.' In R. J. Kleber, C. R. Figley & B. P. Gersons (eds). *Beyond trauma: cultural and societal dynamics*, pp. 17–30. New York: Plenum.

Summerfield, D. 1999. 'A critique of seven assumptions behind psychological trauma programmes in war-affected areas.' *Social Science and Medicine*, 48(10): 1449–62.

Summerfield, D. 2001. 'The invention of post-traumatic stress disorder and the usefulness of a psychiatric category.' *British Medical Journal*, 322(7278): 95–8.

Swart, L., Gilchrist, A., Butchard, A., Seedat, M. & Martin, L. 1999. *Rape surveillance through district surgeons offices in Johannesburg, 1996–1998: evaluation and prevention implications*. Pretoria: Institute of Social and Health Sciences, University of South Africa.

Swartz, L. 1998. *Culture and mental health: a southern African view*. Cape Town: Oxford University Press.

Tedeschi, R. G. & Calhoun, L. G. 2004. Posttraumatic growth: conceptual foundations and empirical evidence. *Psychological Inquiry*, 15(1): 1–18.

Tedeschi, R. G., Calhoun, L. G. & A. McCann. 2007. 'Evaluating resource gain: understanding and misunderstanding posttraumatic growth.' *Applied Psychology: An International Review*, 56(3): 396–406.

Terr, L. 1991. 'Childhood trauma: an outline and overview.' *American Journal of Psychiatry*, 148(1): 10–20.

Thacker, M. 2008. 'Meaning-making amongst South African survivors of violent crime.' Paper presented at the 14th South African Psychology Congress, Johannesburg, August.

Thompson, M. 2000. 'Life after rape: a chance to speak?' *Sexual and Relationship Therapy*, 15(4): 325–43.

True, W. R., Rise, J., Eisen, S., Heath, A. C., Goldberg, J., Lyons, M., Nowak, J. 1993. 'A twin study of genetic and environmental contributions to liability for posttraumatic stress symptoms.' *Archives of General Psychiatry*, 50: 257–64.

Truth and Reconciliation Commission. 1998. *Truth and Reconciliation Commission of South Africa Report, Vol. 1*. Cape Town: CTP.

Truth and Reconciliation Commission. 1998. *Truth and Reconciliation Commission of South Africa Report, Vol. 3*. Cape Town: CTP.

Truth and Reconciliation Commission. 1998. *Truth and Reconciliation Commission of South Africa Report, Vol. 5*. Cape Town: CTP.

Tucker, P. & Trautman, R. 2000. 'Understanding and treating PTSD: past, present and future.' *Bulletin of the Menninger Clinic*, 64(3): 37–52.

Van der kolk, B. A. 1996a. 'Trauma and memory.' In B. A. van der Kolk, A. C. McFarlane & L. Weisaeth (eds). *Traumatic stress: the effects of overwhelming experience on mind, body and society*, pp. 279–302. New York: Guilford Press.

Van der kolk, B. A. 1996*b*. 'The complexity of adaptation to trauma.' In B. A. van der Kolk, A. C. McFarlane & L. Weisaeth (eds). *Traumatic stress: the effects of overwhelming experience on mind, body and society*, pp. 182–213. New York: Guilford Press.

Van Niekerk, A., du Toit, N., Nowell, M. J., Moore, S. & Van As, A. B. 2004. 'Childhood burn injury: epidemiological, management and emerging injury prevention studies.' In S. Suffla, A. van Niekerk & N. Duncan (eds). *Crime, violence and injury prevention in South Africa: developments and challenges*, pp. 145–57. Tygerberg: Medical Research Council-University of South Africa Crime, Violence and Injury Lead Programme.

Van Niekerk, A., Rode, H. & Laflamme, L. 2004. 'Incidence and patterns of childhood burn injuries in the Western Cape, South Africa.' *Burns*, 30(4): 341–7.

Ward, C. L., Flisher, A. J., Zissis, C., Muller, M. & Lombard, C. 2001. 'Exposure to violence and its relationship to psychopathology in adolescents.' *Injury Prevention*, 7(4): 297–301.

Ward, C., Martin, E., Theron, C. & Distiller, B. 2007. 'Factors affecting resilience in children exposed to violence.' *South African Journal of Psychology*, 37(1): 165–87.

Watts, J. & Eagle, G. 2002. 'When objects attack in reality: psychoanalytic contributions to formulations of the impact and treatment of traumatic stress incidences: Part II.' *Psychoanalytic Psychotherapy in South Africa*, 11(1): 8–13.

Wauchope, B. A. & Strauss, M. A. 1990. 'Physical punishment and physical abuse of American children: incidence rates by age, gender and occupational class.' In M. A. Strauss & R. J. Gelles (eds). *Physical violence in American families*, pp. 133–48. New Brunswick, NJ: Transaction Publishers.

Weine, S. M., Kulenovic, A. D., Pavkovic, I. & Gibbons, R. 1998. 'Testimony psychotherapy in Bosnian refugees: a pilot study.' *American Journal of Psychiatry*, 155(12): 1720–6.

Welz, T., Hosegood, V., Jaffar, S., Batzing-Feigenbaum, J., Herbst, K. & Newell, M. 2007. 'Continued very high prevalence of HIV infection in rural KwaZulu-Natal, South Africa: a population-based longitudinal study.' *AIDS*, 21(11): 1467–72.

White, M. & Epston, D. 1990. *Narrative means to therapeutic ends*. New York: W. W. Norton.

Wigren, J. 1994. 'Narrative completion in the treatment of trauma.' *Psychotherapy*, 31(3): 415–23.

Williams, D. R., Herman, A., Kessler, R. C., Sonnega, J., Seedat, S., Stein, D. J., Moomai, H., & Wilson, C. M. 2004. 'The South Africa stress and health study: rationale and design.' *Metabolic Brain Disease*, 19(1-2): 135–47.

Williams, R. & Joseph, S. 1999. 'Conclusions: an integrative psychosocial model of PTSD.' In W. Yule (ed.). *Post-traumatic stress disorders: concepts and therapy*, pp. 297–314. Chichester, England: Wiley.

Williams, S. L., Williams, D. R., Stein, D. J., Seedat, S., Jackson, P. B. & Moomal, H. 2007. 'Multiple traumatic events and psychological distress: The South Africa Stress and Health Study.' *Journal of Traumatic Stress*, 20(5): 845–55.

Wilson, J. P. 1994. 'The historical evolution of PTSD diagnostic criteria: from Freud to DSM-IV.' *Journal of Traumatic Stress*, 7 (3): 681–98.

Wilson, J. P. & Moran, T. A. 1998. 'Psychological trauma: post traumatic stress disorder and spirituality.' *Journal of Psychology and Theology*, 26(2): 168–78.

Wilson, J. P. & Lindy, J. D. 1999. 'Empathic strain and countertransference.' In M. J. Horowitz (ed.). *Essential papers on posttraumatic stress disorder*, pp. 518–43. New

York: New York University Press.

World Health Organisation. 1992. *The ICD-10 classification of mental and behavioural disorders: clinical descriptions and diagnostic guidelines*. Geneva: WHO.

Wyatt, G. E., Guthrie, D. & Notgrass, C. M. 1992. 'Differential effects of women's child sexual abuse and subsequent sexual revictimisation.' *Journal of Consulting and Clinical Psychology*, 60(2): 167–73.

Yehuda, R. 1999. 'Biological factors associated with susceptibility to posttraumatic stress disorder.' *Canadian Journal of Psychiatry*, 44(1): 21–32.

Yehuda, R. 2000. 'Neuroendocrinology.' In D. Nutt, J. R. T. Davidson & J. Zohar (eds). *Post-traumatic stress disorder: diagnosis, management and treatment*, pp. 53–68. London: Martin Dunitz.

Young, A. 1995. *The harmony of illusions: inventing posttraumatic stress disorder*. New Jersey: Princeton University Press.

Yule, W. 2003. 'Early intervention strategies with traumatised children, adolescents and families.' In R. Orner & U. Schnyder (eds). *Reconstructing early interventions after trauma*, pp. 25–50. Oxford: Oxford University Press.

Yule, W., Perrin, S. & Smith, P. 1999. 'Post-traumatic stress disorders in children and adolescents.' In W. Yule (ed.). *Post-traumatic stress disorders: concepts and therapy*, pp. 25–50. Chichester; John Wiley and Sons.

Zlotnick, C., Johnson, J., Kohn, R., Vicente, B., Rioseco, P. & Saldivia, S. 2006. 'Epidemiology of trauma, post-traumatic stress disorder (PTSD) and co-morbid disorders in Chile.' *Psychological Medicine*, 36(11): 1523–33.

Zoellner, T. & Maercker, A. 2006. 'Posttraumatic growth in clinical psychology: a critical review and introduction of a two-component model.' *Clinical Psychology Review*, 26(5): 626–53.

Zungu-Dirwayi, N., Kaminer, D., Mbanga, I. & Stein, D. J. 2004. 'The psychiatric sequelae of human rights violations: a challenge for primary health care.' *Journal of Nervous and Mental Disease*, 192(4): 255–9.

ABOUT THE AUTHORS

Debra Kaminer is a senior lecturer in the Department of Psychology at the University of Cape Town. She conducted her doctoral dissertation on the psychological effects of giving testimony to the Truth and Reconciliation Commission, while based at the Medical Research Council's Unit on Anxiety and Stress Disorders. She has also published journal articles and book chapters, and presented conference papers, in the areas of childhood trauma and PTSD, the link between different forms of violence and PTSD in the South African population, and the use of testimony and trauma narratives in interventions with survivors. In addition to her research, she has counselled trauma survivors in her own clinical practice, supervised the clinical work of trainee psychologists working with traumatised adults and children, and provided consultation for a number of volunteer organisations that work with trauma survivors. She is currently conducting research aimed at documenting the knowledge accumulated by trauma counsellors and clinicians in South Africa.

Gillian Eagle is a professor of Psychology in the School of Human and Community Development at the University of the Witwatersrand. She has worked in the traumatic stress field as researcher, clinician and activist over a period of about twenty-five years. She has offered counselling, training, supervision and consulting services to a range of non-governmental organisations working in the trauma field, including People Opposing Women Abuse (POWA), Durban Rape Crisis, the Organisation for Appropriate Social Services in South Africa (OASSSA), the National Peace Accord Trust (NPAT), the South Africa Institute for Traumatic Stress (SAITS) and the Centre for the Study of Violence and Reconciliation (CSVR). Her doctorate was on the experiences of men who had been victims of violent crime and she has supervised a number of research studies in the traumatic stress field. She has presented at several international and national conferences and published journal articles and book chapters on a range of topics relating to traumatic stress. Although her interest in the field is broad, she has a particular interest in attributional, gender-related and socio-political aspects of trauma. She continues to work in the area of traumatic stress as both clinician and researcher.

INDEX

Please note: Page numbers in italics refer to Figures, Tables and Boxes.

Printed and bound by CPI Group (UK) Ltd, Croydon, CR0 4YY

16/04/2025

14658441-0001